In Time of Plague

IN TIME OF PLAGUE

The History and Social Consequences of Lethal Epidemic Disease

Edited by Arien Mack

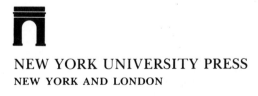

NEW YORK UNIVERSITY PRESS
NEW YORK AND LONDON

Library of Congress Cataloging-in-Publication Data
In time of plague : the history and social consequences of lethal
epidemic disease / edited by Arien Mack.
p. cm.
Includes index.
ISBN 0-8147-5467-8
1. Epidemics—History. 2. Epidemiology—Social aspects. 3. AIDS
(Disease)—Social aspects. I. Mack, Arien.
RA649.I5   1991
306.4′61—dc20   91-13750
                                                                CIP

c 10 9 8 7 6 5 4 3 2 1

New York University Press books are printed on acid-free paper,
and their binding materials are chosen for strength and durability.

Contents

Foreword

Wᴡʀɪᴛɪɴɢ of London's plague-ridden summer of 1592 in his *Summer's Last Will and Testament,* the poet, novelist and pamphleteer Thomas Nashe gave the stanzas of his famous litany a refrain from the English Prayer Book's office for the dead:

> Adieu, farewell earth's bliss,
> This world uncertain is;
> Fond are life's lustful joys,
> Death proves them all but toys,
> None from his darts can fly,
> I am sick, I must die.
>   Lord, have mercy on us!
>
> Rich men, trust not in wealth,
> Gold cannot by you health;
> Physic himself must fade,
> All things to end are made.
> The plague full swift goes by.
> I am sick, I must die.
>   Lord, have mercy on us!

We are now in time of plague. But this time it is during a period of our historical consciousness which would seem to have put the very term "plague," and the realms of ignorance that it signifies for our general knowledge of the etiology of infectious disease, far behind us. The word itself has come to be used in two principle ways. The first designates the epidemic infections by *bacillus pestis* in its various bubonic, pneumonic and septicaemic forms that started to overrun Europe in the fourteenth century, and still manifests for the medical and historial layman an aura of factual rats and lice cloaked by superstitious fiction.

Our other use of "plague" is that of the older and basic term, the biblical and proverbial one, referring to the ten disasters with which the Lord smote the Egyptians in Exodus. Of these, at most two, the boils and the murrain decimating the livestock —anthrax, hoof-and-mouth, or whatever—were infectious diseases, or in any way like "plague" in the first sense; generally, they comprised a series of graded horrors, from pests through pestilence, through darkness and significantly selective death, which *struck* (and this is the operative word) the Egyptians. For our English word "plague," is derived from the Latin *plaga* which means a blow, a wound, the mark left by something striking one: something with which one has been stricken. It quite rightly translates the Hebrew word for the ten plagues, *maggefot,* which similarly derives from the root *neggef,* or blow. (The word for contagious illness is *dever,* and is used only of one of the plagues, the "pestilence." This is translated by the Latin *pestis,* a word, like infectious disease itself until the nineteenth century, "of obscure origin.") The etymological implication of "plague" privileges the world of the patient, the sufferer, rather than that of the healer, interpreter or understander. A plague is what one has been assaulted with. And when that is some bodily harm seeming to develop from within one, it is rather an *illness* (as the medical anthropologist Arthur Kleinman has distinguished them) than a *disease*—a condition possessed of the sufferer, rather than a conceptual construction of biomedicine.

It is to the Greek historian Thucydides that we owe our canonical analytic account of *pestis,* of "lethal epidemic disease" in the language of this volume's subtitle. His chronicle of the epidemic *(loimos)*—of still disputed biomedical character—that struck the Athenians during the Peloponnesian War is exemplary in its description of the effects of widespread, uncontrollable infectious disease upon the life of the *polis* and, indeed, upon institutions of hope and fear, as in his famous observation that (in Rex Warner's translation) "As for the gods, it seemed to be the same thing whether one worshipped them or

not, when one saw the good and the bad dying indiscrimi-
nately." It is also to Thucydides that we owe a notion of the
moral consequences of plagues, one reciprocal to that of their
moral causes, as in the case of the biblical plagues as God's
willed blows of retribution.

Medical science might be said to have come, since the middle
of the nineteenth century, to have disinfected the first meaning, that of a specific *pestis*, from contamination by the connotations of *plaga*, the second one. With the very identification of
a microbe, together with its vectors of transmission, as the
"causes" of the disease, the Divine or otherwise ineffable deliverer—and mode of delivery—of the plague with which one is
stricken became a matter of myth and, in its decayed or institutionalized form, catastrophic popular error. We have never
been entirely free of the feeling that *pestis* is *plaga*. Any individual person, no matter how rational, is bound to have a private
sense of his or her own illness, whatever it may be. More
generally, those of us over a certain age can remember when,
in the United States, poliomyelitis was still something of an
endemic summer plague, spottily dispensed—for all practical
purposes—by Fortune. From the point of view of the individual imagination and of the individual illness, cancer, while not
communicably infectious, is in its own way epidemic in a plague-
like way. All of us feel our illnesses—even those of annoyance,
like the common cold—as *plagae*, as blows with which we have
been struck. And yet, of course, nobody, and nothing, has
delivered them. But for the most part, the concept of *pestis* as
plaga we have tended to consign to an earlier world-picture or
episteme.

It is precisely because of the crucial threat, and the complex
social ramifications, of the epidemic spread of the HIV virus in
the last decades of the twentieth century that we can feel again
how "the plague full swift goes by." But it is generally because
of our growing realization that we are no longer able, thanks
to three centuries of enlightenment, to feel ourselves delivered

from a specific aspect of how "this would uncertain is," that it
has seemed necessary to open up again the book of plague.
Our private, personal superstitions and our hopes for being
able to dispel them had shifted, it seemed, from the realm of
deadly contagious disease to those of perhaps deeper biochemical mysteries. But now we are reminded of such matters as
those of personal infectiousness, of rights and responsibilities
of the ill and the healthy at a moment in American history
when so much vox populi seems to harp on individual rights
and entitlements but only on public responsibilities, on how
much or how little my neighbor's disease may be, or may be
said to be, mine, and so many more. And it is altogether
appropriate for us to acknowledge that we have lost a good bit
of our conceptual world's certainty, and to proceed to apply to
our new confusion some of what, in those same three centuries,
we have indeed gained.

Contributors

CHARLES E. ROSENBERG is Janice and Julian Bers Professor of the History and Sociology of Science at the University of Pennsylvania and author of *The Care of Strangers: The Rise of America's Hospital System.*

WILLIAM H. FOEGE is Executive Director of the Carter Center in Atlanta.

JOSHUA LEDERBERG, a 1958 Nobel laureate, is president emeritus of Rockefeller University.

DOROTHY NELKIN is university professor of sociology at New York University, the author of *Selling Science: How the Press Covers Science and Technology,* and co-author of *The Animal Rights Crusade: The Growth of a Moral Protest.*

SANDER L. GILMAN is Goldwin Smith Professor of Humane Studies at Cornell University, the coeditor, with Steven T. Katz, of *Anti-Semitism in Times of Crisis* (New York University Press), and the author of *Disease and Representation: Images of Illness from Madness to AIDS.*

LEWIS THOMAS, president emeritus of the Memorial Sloan-Kettering Cancer Center in New York City, is currently a scholar in residence at Cornell University Medical College.

BARBARA GUTMANN ROSENKRANTZ is professor of the history of science at Harvard University and author of *Public Health and the State.*

BARUCH S. BLUMBERG, a 1976 Nobel laureate, is professor of medicine and anthropology at Balliol College, Oxford, England.

ALLAN M. BRANDT is associate professor in the department of social medicine at the University of North Carolina and the author of *No Magic Bullet: A Social History of Venereal Disease in the United States since 1880*.

PAUL SLACK is a fellow and tutor in modern history at Exeter College, Oxford and author of *Poverty and Policy in Tudor and Stuart England*.

GEORGE KATEB is professor of politics at Princeton University and author of *Hannah Arendt: Politics, Conscience, Evil*.

RICHARD POIRIER is Marius Bewley Professor of English at Rutgers University, editor of *Raritan Quarterly*, and author of *The Renewal of Literature*.

ANTHONY QUINTON is a former president of Trinity College, Oxford, a former chairman of the British Library, and author of *Thought and Thinkers*.

DAVID A. J. RICHARDS is professor of law at New York University and author of *Toleration and the Constitution* and *Foundations of American Constitutionalism*.

Introduction

BY ARIEN MACK

THIS diverse collection of essays represents an attempt to set the recent and alarming outbreak of AIDS in perspective by considering it in the context of the social history of past lethal epidemics. The focus of attention is on the many ways in which diseases, particularly catastrophic infections and contagious diseases, are socially as well as biologically defined. This emphasis is meant to lead to the recognition that diseases are not simple biological entities which belong to the exclusive domain of scientists and physicians. They are social-cultural events as much as biological and medical ones, and so coming to terms with them cannot simply be a matter of waving the scientist's magic wand.

The choice of so ominous and threatening a title as *In Time of Plague* was deliberate and based on at least two reasons. First, for good or ill, the word "plague" effectively captures the emotional associations frequently engendered by reports about AIDS. The word acknowledges the unfamiliar fears it has awakened. After decades of dividing our time between apocalyptic fears of nuclear holocaust and private fears of personal ruin, we now face a threat that is profoundly social, requiring a public, community response. Most of us until recently have assumed, perhaps without thinking, that the number of life-threatening infectious diseases was finite, soon to be cured and prevented by medical science. So the study of plagues was delegated exclusively to medical and social historians. Now it appears that this idea that we stand outside our own history, that we, unlike our forebears, are immune to widespread medical disasters, is very doubtful.

The word "plague" appears in the title for a more specific

reason as well. Its presence points the way to the problem that must be addressed. In fact, the problem we face can be seen in the very considerations that made the word seem appropriate, for the exotic connotations of the term exercise their influence over our emotions, even when the word itself is not spoken. The fact is that the past is both too much and too little with us in our public deliberations about AIDS; its images of disease affect us precisely because we so rarely take them into account. The hope is that these scholarly discussions will allow our present and our past to speak with each other. With luck they may permit us to discern the similarities between our past and our present, untangle overlooked differences, and reflect on how we should now act.

The essays in this book are divided into four sections. The first section, "The Definition and Control of Disease," is concerned with a group of related questions:

(a) How has the definition of disease differed in different historical moments? Are there cultural invariants that determine how diseases are perceived or defined? How does the definition of disease as a consequence of behavior, the presence of some biological process, or as the manifestation of a particular set of symptoms affect the social response?

(b) How have new technologies, advances in the science of epidemiology and mass information gathering changed our perception and response to disease? Under that circumstances has it been deemed appropriate, or is it appropriate, to control information or behavior? For example, when has quarantine been appropriate or effective?

(c) What problems follow from reporting the results of medical research to the public?

The second section contains only one paper. This paper by Lewis Thomas, "Science and Health: Possibilities, Probabilities, and Limitations," presents an optimistic view of what the future of medical science promises us.

The third section, "Case Histories," contains three papers, two of which recount the social histories of earlier plagues, the Black Death and syphilis, while the remaining paper, by Baruch Blumberg, tells the story of hepatitis B and the search for a preventive vaccine.

The three papers in the last section, "Moral Dilemmas," concern the thicket of moral problems raised by the presence of lethal, contagious diseases. What norms should govern our thinking about responsibility, culpability, legality, and confidentiality? What does society owe the victims? What are the responsibilities of the carrier population? How do we deal with the patient's right to privacy in the face of the physician's duty to warn and the public's right to know?

These papers at their best illustrate how much there is to be learned from a colloquy among scientists, social scientists, and philosophers, all of whom are concerned with common problems.

The original versions of these papers were presented at a *Social Research* conference held at the New School for Social Research in 1988 and the papers appeared in the Autumn 1988 issue of the journal. The conference was made possible by the generous support of the Rockefeller Foundation and the Edna McConnell Clark Foundation for which I am extremely grateful. The initial plans for this conference emerged at a planning meeting in the fall of 1986 attended by Gert H. Brieger, William H. Welch Professor of the History of Medicine, Johns Hopkins; John Hollander, poet and professor of English at Yale University; Shirley Lindenbaum, anthropologist and colleague at the Graduate Faculty of the New School; Dorothy Nelkin, professor, Program on Science, Technology and Society, Cornell University, currently Clare Boothe Luce Visiting Professor, Department of Sociology, New York University; Kenneth Prewitt, political scientist and vice president of the Rockefeller Foundation; Susan Sontag, novelist and critic; Paul Starr, sociologist and professor at Princeton University;

Jamie Walkup, editorial associate and co-organizer of the conference, and myself.

The idea for this project was first suggested by my cherished friend, John Hollander. My valued colleague, Jamie Walkup, collaborated with me in its development every step of the way. I am especially grateful to them both.

I. The Definition and Control of Disease—An Introduction

BY CHARLES E. ROSENBERG

AIDS has reminded us of some very old truths, truths most Americans had managed to forget during the past four decades. Epidemic infectious disease is not simply a historical phenomenon—or one limited like famine to the nonwhite in remote continents. By the end of the 1970s, most Americans had come to regard themselves as no longer at risk; infectious disease was almost by definition amenable to medical intervention. Not since the last severe polio threats more than a quarter century ago has the United States experienced the collective fear of epidemic disease.[1]

AIDS has helped us remember some other things as well. One is the way in which epidemic disease mobilizes widespread social response to the same stimulus; because AIDS was new to the 1980s that response was particularly intense and illuminating. Our reactions have underlined both our common humanity and America's cultural and institutional diversity. Epidemics serve as natural sampling devices, mirrors held up to society in which more general patterns of social values and attitudes appear in sharp relief. AIDS has demonstrated as well the way in which epidemics take place at a number of levels—biological event, social perception, collective response,

[1] Influenza does not seem to have the same ability to inspire widespread fear—in part because we have also forgotten the 1918 flu epidemic.

and, finally, the individual, the existential and moral. Yet these several aspects of an epidemic can be disaggregated only for the purpose of analysis, for they are intricately linked and constantly interactive. Each disease entity, as a social phenomenon, is a uniquely configured cluster of events and responses in both the biological and social spheres. AIDS reminds us not only of the multiple levels at which disease exists, but the urgent need to understand the interactions between these constituent aspects of the phenomenon we call an epidemic. The following papers focus differentially, in fact, on those levels, Lederberg emphasizing the biological, Foege organized public policy, Nelkin and Gilman the individual and attitudinal. Finally, AIDS has made it clear that we are not masters of life; there are limits built not only into humankind's genetic makeup but into our changing ecological relationship with the rest of the world and the multiplicity of organisms that inhabit it.

We tend to think of ills as either fundamentally biological and unambiguous in their medical identity (rooted in a well-understood biopathological mechanism) or as value-laden and problematic in their relationship to medical models and medical authority. AIDS occupies a position at both ends of that spectrum; it is an affect-laden occasion for the blaming of victims while, at the same time, it is the consequence of a particular and extraordinarily deadly biological mechanism.[2] This new pestilence can hardly be considered an arbitrary exercise in the labeling of deviance.

It is a plague in the classic sense, allied to such predecessors as bubonic plague, yellow fever, and cholera. Joshua Lederberg's essay construes AIDS as pathobiological process and humankind as animal, subject to the ultimately unpredictable vagaries of its physical and biological environment. By invoking the logically linked contributions of Darwin and

[2] I have discussed these issues in greater detail in "Disease and Social Order in America: Perceptions and Expectations," *Milbank Quarterly* 64, Suppl. 1 (1986): 34–55.

Pasteur, Lederberg seeks to place his argument in a cosmic framework, in which man's cognitive capacities are but one variable in a complex, ever-changing, and unpredictable universe. When he alludes to the microbiological events that have taken place in his laboratory test tube, Lederberg refers metaphorically to man's place on earth—our particular test tube, in which human population has increased rapidly and perhaps ominously in the past century.

Dorothy Nelkin and Sander Gilman focus on a rather different level: the way in which men and women have tended to reduce their sense of vulnerability in times of plague by defining others as the ailment's appropriate and likely victims—creating reassuring frameworks in which to control and disarm otherwise disconcerting realities. Cultural values and social location have always provided the materials for self-serving constructions of epidemiological risk. The poor, the alien, the sinner have all served as convenient objects for such stigmatizing speculations.

William Foege's essay emphasizes a rather more public and institutionalized response to epidemic disease. Public health is a contested terrain in which objective data interact with such factors as the status of physicians and assumptions about state power. The relationship between knowledge and its application is always subject to negotiation; every historian of public health is well aware of this disconcerting reality. The brief history of AIDS has illustrated this truth with disheartening clarity.

But if AIDS illustrates timeless themes, it suggests some aspects of novelty as well. The pace of change in the late twentieth century is intense—as exemplified, for example, in the rapidity with which air travel helped spread the virus or the speed with which modern laboratories identified this new clinical entity and demonstrated its cause. Other institutions, too, have shaped perception and response in novel patterns. The state and its several agencies, for example, as well as print and electronic media have played significant roles in shaping the response of a diverse and fragmented society. We have available to us an array of policy and attitudinal choices vastly different from those available to Europeans when they encountered plague in the fourteenth century or cholera in the nineteenth.

But for many Americans the ultimate meaning of AIDS must be moral. The precise lesson to be drawn from the history of AIDS will differ, just as Americans differ among themselves in their religious and social orientations. I was particularly struck in this connection with the resonant image of Joshua Lederberg's test tube. The ultimate moral implicit in this metaphor would have been clear enough to that dauntless Massachusetts pioneer in public health, Cotton Mather. We are all sinners in a test tube, he might have observed, in the hands of an awesome and possibly angry God whose acts transcend man's capacity for understanding.

Plagues: Perceptions of Risk and Social Responses

BY WILLIAM H. FOEGE

POLYBIUS taught us, over 2000 years ago, that the world is an organic whole,[1] where everything affects everything. Plagues demonstrate that truth—crossing cultures, crossing time, but also joining cultures and time inextricably, influencing the births and deaths of people, careers, and nations. Indeed, in a recently overworked phrase, "plagues bend history."

Perhaps rivaling the Black Death, which has received so much attention, was the pandemic of cholera which broke the boundaries of India in the early nineteenth century, moved across Russia by 1830, caused havoc at Mecca in 1831, moved across Europe in 1831 and 1832, arrived in the United States and went by canal boat to Albany and then to the Missouri River by 1833, where it became the determining factor for many wagon trains over the next years. In 1835, Marcus Whitman, the first medical missionary to the American west, made his initial journey to Oregon and was credited with saving a wagon train by stopping a cholera outbreak.[2] That epidemic allowed him to earn his reputation and start a career. Twelve years later, another epidemic, this one of measles, led

[1] Polybius, Bk. I, pp. 3–4 (ca. 150 B.C.).
[2] Bernard DeVoto, *Across the Wide Missouri* (Boston: Houghton Mifflin, 1947), p. 220.

to the Whitman Mission massacre, ending his career and the lives of the mission personnel.[3]

The Whitman Mission story becomes a paradigm for what has happened across cultures and nations. In the early eighteenth century, British troops began to receive variolation with smallpox virus, after Lady Montagu introduced the practice she had observed in Turkey, where her husband was ambassador.[4] Fifty years later, the battle of Quebec, where American troops outnumbered the British two to one, was lost by American troops when smallpox swept through their ranks but spared the British troops who had been variolated. (Some Canadians to this day worship smallpox as the deliverer from United States citizenship.)

In 1801, Thomas Jefferson acquired smallpox vaccine and personally administered it to his family and neighbors at Monticello. In 1804, he gave vaccine to Lewis and Clark, instructing them to administer it to Indians because of their high mortality rates due to smallpox. But it was too little and smallpox opened the west, decimating tribes and breaking their spirit. DeVoto writes about the 1837 outbreak, "All summer long not a single Indian came to Fort McKenzie. . . . Early in the fall Culbertson set out to . . . find out what was wrong. . . . Then at the Three Forks he found a village. No sound came from it as he approached, there were no horses or dogs, no children, no uproar. Presently they smelled the stench and then 'hundreds of decaying forms of human beings . . . lay scattered everywhere among the lodges.' "[5] On July 14 a young Mandan died of smallpox. Six months later only a hundred of the 1600 Mandans were still alive and no tribal organization could be maintained. There are no full-blooded Mandans today.

What lessons have we learned from this continuous flow of

[3] *Ibid.*, pp. 371–372.
[4] Donald R. Hopkins, *Princes and Peasants: Smallpox in History* (Chicago: University of Chicago Press, 1983), pp. 47–49.
[5] *Ibid.*, p. 291.

plague history? Are we truly better off because of what has happened upstream, or do the problems continue to change so dramatically that the lessons are only marginally beneficial? In this first session, we can only touch on some of the lessons of plague history. My attempts will be modest—to say something about:

   (a) the definition of plagues
   (b) the perception of risk
   (c) responses

Definition

The definition of plague offered by the 1986 *Webster Medical Desk Dictionary,* describing plague as an epidemic disease causing a high rate of mortality, is inadequate for several reasons. Epidemiologists now commonly use the term *epidemic* to describe an unusual occurrence of a disease or condition. Thus, while a single case of smallpox would constitute an epidemic, the million cases of gonorrhea each year in the United States would be considered an endemic disease but not necessarily an epidemic.

Therefore, two problems with *Webster's* definition of the term are particularly significant. First, plagues do not have to be epidemic: a plague can be endemic, a constant presence. Second, mortality rates should not be the criterion for measurement. In describing one plague, the Old Testament notes the presence of fiery serpents, now known to be Dracunculiasis, or Guinea worm. This disease is associated with low mortality, yet anyone who has seen this ugly, debilitating scourge of poor areas knows it is a plague.

In fact, the definition of plague continues to change. We can all accept that smallpox, yellow fever, and cholera have been major plagues of history. But, in the last ten years, our society has legitimately expanded the definition of plague to recognize a plague of ancient and major proportions—that is, violence. Historically, the two major causes of premature mortality have been infectious diseases and violence. The violence plague resisted the best efforts of science, religion, and law until very recently. To characterize it as a plague appears accurate.

Other, newer uses of the word *plague* involve chemicals. The agent need not be a microorganism but can be a chemical such as benzene or kepone, which can produce acute or chronic illness. Also, it is now common to speak of a lung-cancer plague, an outbreak or plague of strokes or coronary occlusion. Since the use of the word has enlarged, perhaps a better working definition would be "a disease or other condition causing high mortality *or* morbidity and often accompanied by social dislocation."

Perception of Risk

The response to a plague or threat of a plague is in some ways dependent on the perception of risk held by individuals and decision-makers. The perception can be quite different for the same disease depending on whether it is endemic or epidemic. For example, twenty-five years ago, in the state of Bihar, India, smallpox was endemic. Year in and year out it caused devastating illness and a large number of deaths. It was a scourge to be feared, but it did not cause panic primarily because explanations for the disease were incorporated into the culture and this provided acceptance and perhaps even a fatalistic attitude. At the same time, in Africa, smallpox would infect a given geographic area only periodically. Writings of anthropologists indicate that in some cases this would result in panic, the flight of a village population, and extensive social disruption.

We know from recent studies that the perception of risk that people have for many conditions is unrealistic, unstable, and influenced by illusions of control. For example, people have some concept that microorganisms entail different risks, and the fear of the AIDS virus is totally different from the fear of strep throat. But at the same time we bring far less discrimination to chemical risks. For many, chemical risks are blurred, with saccharin, nitrites, and cigarettes having similar risks.

These studies have also found that the amount of control felt by a person greatly changes the perception of risk. People will accept high risks with cigarette smoking, fast driving, drug use, and other similar activities if they have control of placing themselves at risk. But they will reject even small or nonexistent risks, such as with food additives, fluoridation, or radiation if they feel they have no control over the exposure.

This has undoubtedly been a factor in the perception of and response to plagues in the past. People who thought they had some control over their own destinies reacted in different ways. This could have played a role in the continuing flow of Europeans to West Africa in the nineteenth century, despite known endemic plague conditions such as yellow fever and malaria that exacted major tolls. We know that mortality rates were very high for early Europeans in West Africa. Mungo Park, a physician, led an expedition attempting to map the Niger River. Within a few months all but six of his men had died of disease. The last six drowned when their boat capsized.

As we learn from *Ladder of Bones,* missionaries may have felt a divine calling, but early traders accepted such plague risks because of the money involved and the knowledge that if they survived for one year they would be placed in supervisory positions.[6] They must have felt a degree of control which led them to the conviction that they were survivors.

The same phenomenon was operating when the early mountain men of 160 years ago went west. Their annual rendezvous made it clear that in some years over 50 percent of

---

[6] Ellen Thorp, *Ladder of Bones* (Great Britain: Fontana Books, 1966).

the newcomers died, and yet their belief that they were in control caused them to accept such risks.

The same phenomenon occurs with modern plagues. A recent article by Ken Warner gives the Las Vegas odds for smokers. The net effect of freeing our society from all tobacco mortality would be a life-expectancy increase of one to two years. The average gain for smokers would be four to five years. But not all smokers die because of tobacco, and therefore for the smoker who actually experiences a tobacco-related death the loss is approximately fifteen years.[7] Subjecting oneself to such a plague requires either a strong feeling of control that will allow one to beat the odds or a strong sense of fatalism with no ability to alter the future.

The same is seen with AIDS, where some feel no threat even in the face of high-risk behavior while others feel no control even in the absence of risk. Episodes such as we have seen in Arcadia, Florida, result from many converging vectors, including feelings of vulnerability, no control, scientific illiteracy in interpreting the data, and lack of confidence in the authorities who indicated that these children did not present a risk.

Response

A watershed event in plague history was the point when individuals or groups moved from fatalistic acceptance to nonfatalistic action. Whether that action was effective is a separate question, but action is an old response in most cultures. In West Africa, fetishers intervened on behalf of smallpox victims. They would explain to smallpox victims what they must do to appease the gods. If the patient lived, the fetisher could take the credit and receive the appropriate

[7] Kenneth E. Warner, "Health and Economic Implications of a Tobacco-free Society," *Journal of the American Medical Association* 258 (1987): 2080.

rewards. If the patient died, the fetisher would explain how the patient had failed to carry out the recommended actions.

From Africa to India, to the Soviet Union, to Western Europe, religious ceremonies, beliefs, and activities developed to intervene, to appease the smallpox deity in order to reduce the intensity of this plague. The use of the color red, for example, in fighting smallpox seems to have been common and practiced in diverse parts of the world. Whether there was a common origin to this practice that spread through trade and travel or whether it has a multifocal origin is unknown. Even in modern times, we still engage in symbolism in our desire to appease the deities, whether keeping innocent and harmless children with positive HIV tests out of school or staying out of drafts to avoid the cold virus.

Social Regression. Today, we have experts to comment on the social implications of plague. But it is important to note that in general it has been easier for society to get answers in the area of biology and chemistry than in the areas of sociology, law, and ethics. We have, for instance, found it less difficult to develop a test for HIV antibodies than to develop guidelines on how to use that test. Likewise it is easier to develop vaccines than to get societies to use them. The stress of a plague compounds the problem, and social regression has been a common effect of disease outbreaks in the past. From the mistreatment of individuals to the total breakdown of social interactions, disease outbreaks have distorted society.

This unfortunate trend continues with AIDS. At the individual level, old and new prejudices have surfaced. Most gay men would happily return to the social acceptance of 1980 rather than face the ostracism that the AIDS crisis has produced in the last three years. Haitians have had difficulty in securing jobs, and some countries require testing of foreign students. Tourism in Africa has been adversely affected, and while the lesson that we are citizens of one globe should be the predominant one to arise from this pandemic, instead AIDS is causing social fragmentation throughout many cultures. A recent editorial in *Science* said, "We have our problems today but at least we are not burning witches to stop the spread of disease."[8] Perhaps, but our actions are just as primitive.

Effective Intervention. Contrary to what we might expect, effective intervention is not all recent and often cannot be attributed to a single social group, much less an individual. The isolation or quarantine of smallpox cases to prevent spread was practiced long before quarantine procedures were used by governments. In West Africa, villagers would build a hut outside of the village for the isolation of smallpox cases. Food and care would be entrusted to a person who had already recovered from the disease.

Variolation, or the use of smallpox virus (not cowpox or vaccinia virus), was developed as a successful intervention tool thousands of years ago in China, India, and Africa. It was an effective, empirically developed intervention that was eventually used throughout the world.

But it was Edward Jenner who, 192 years ago, changed the history of intervention by developing a plague-prevention tool that involved small risk, was easy to use, and was very effective. Poets had noted the nice complexions of milkmaids, but it required Jenner to ask the scientific questions whether that was true and, if so, why? This line of questioning led him to develop smallpox vaccine. Despite its many advantages, however, it took the world 181 years to fully capitalize on this development. The fact that we have gone over ten years without a case of smallpox should embolden us to vigorously attack other plagues.

Lessons in application have multiplied dramatically since that time. Semmelweiss taught us the importance of observation and careful analysis of the facts about disease transmission. He carefully noted the disparity between maternal

[8] Daniel E. Koshland, Jr., "The Epidemiology Issue," *Science*, Nov. 21, 1986.

mortality rates on one ward versus another and concluded that the doctors themselves were responsible by examining women after they were involved in performing autopsies. His solution, washing of hands between the two activities, is a monument to simplicity. As Emerson observed, one should avoid over-analysis since often the causes are quite superficial. John Snow also used observation as a tool in the 1850s, and his analysis led him to reach new conclusions about the transmission of cholera, conclusions that were used within decades around the world.

But perhaps the most important step in the response to plagues has not been the dramatic interventions of Semmel-weiss, Snow, and others, but rather the much more mundane development of successful delivery systems. The "institutional-izing" of response techniques so that they are available to everyone and for every plague is a very recent innovation in the history of plague study and control. While the philosophi-cal basis for public health is social justice, the scientific foundation for public health is epidemiology. Although epidemiology was not institutionalized as an academic subject until almost seven decades ago, when Wade Hampton Frost was detailed from the U.S. Public Health Service to establish a department of epidemiology at Johns Hopkins, it is now one of the foundation stones of every school of public health.

But it was not until 1949 that epidemiology became institutionalized in the practice of public health. In that year, Alex Langmuir went from Johns Hopkins to the Communica-ble Disease Center in Atlanta (thereby returning the loan the Public Health Service had made in the form of Wade Hampton Frost) and established the Epidemic Intelligence Service. The techniques he established are now used as standards, not only in the United States but throughout the world.

Langmuir also developed practical systems of surveillance— fundamental for epidemiological analysis—to collect on a routine basis the needed numerators and denominators.

Surprisingly, this country had no nationwide surveillance system for any disease until 1950. In that year a malaria-surveillance program was started, only to find that malaria had quietly disappeared from the country in the 1940s. The next national surveillance program was started for polio during the crisis of the Cutter vaccine incident of 1955. Now there are literally dozens of such systems.

A second important component of the surveillance system is the ability to analyze the information collected in order to define the outbreak or situation and to characterize the extent of disease, the determinants, and the effects. It was such routine analysis that characterized the early days of the AIDS epidemic, and epidemiological analysis predicted the impending problems with blood products. Reviewing the 1983 recommendations on AIDS control, it is evident that the major facts were clearly apparent, because of epidemiology, before a virus was ever isolated. Those 1983 recommendations identified the means of sexual and blood-product transmission and what could be done to prevent transmission.

A third component of the system is the reporting of information back to health departments, other government agencies, academic facilities, and to the public on a weekly basis, which allows everyone to make their own interpretations if they wish. In order to effect the necessary changes in behavior, the public must be able to trust health leadership and must be provided with the most complete and factual information possible. But are there exceptions to sharing information? Obviously, one should not needlessly hurt people, and it should be apparent that the usual medical confidentiality and respect for an individual's privacy are required if we are to retain the cooperation of the public in outbreak investigations.

Such collection, analysis, and response is not new. It is the essence of the examples given earlier with Snow and others. Indeed, even the Whitman massacre was due to the logical collection of data, the correct interpretation that the measles outbreak being experienced by the Indians was due to the Whitman Mission attracting visitors, and the apparently logical intervention of getting rid of the mission.

What is new about the surveillance techniques established by Alex Langmuir is that they were set up to provide *ongoing* evaluations of disease conditions and systematic responses. In the 1960s and 1970s, the same systematic approaches were used around the world for smallpox, and consequently surveillance and epidemiology have become effective tools in most countries.

While we have had an accumulated benefit from all of the various discoveries, the most important lesson of plague history is the value of systematizing our generic approaches to disease control. Second, the lessons of plague history include the need for a surveillance system to accurately define the outbreak, its determinants, distribution, and effects. Third, constant and competent analysis is required to determine the vulnerable points and to develop appropriate interventions. Fourth, responses require providing information to all who need to know, including the general public, and the initiation of public and private control activities.

In conclusion, as bad as the AIDS epidemic is, think what it would have been like fifty or even a hundred years ago, before we had a national surveillance system, before we had the massive educational possibilities of television, before we had the technology for testing to protect the supply of blood products, and before we had a global health leadership in the form of the World Health Organization.

We can take comfort from the lessons learned and at the same time recognize we haven't moved forward adequately in all areas. For example, last year for the first time in thirty-nine years, the United States defaulted on its payment to the World Health Organization, thereby weakening the global effort to control disease. This was not a scientific failure; it was a leadership failure. And it will come back to haunt us.

For all of our scientific advances, we will continue to face plagues forever, and we must now put as much attention on developing our social, legal, and ethical capacities as we have our technical and scientific capacities. To invoke the words of Sir William Osler, "Our mission is of the highest and the noblest kind, not alone in curing disease but in educating the people in the laws of health and in preventing the spread of plagues and pestilence." That is our goal.

Pandemic as a Natural Evolutionary Phenomenon

BY JOSHUA LEDERBERG

My main thesis is that the progress of medical science during the last century has obscured the human species' continued vulnerability to large-scale infection. We fail to acknowledge our relationship to microbes as a *continued* evolutionary process. This is far from equilibrium, and we cannot take for granted near-term outcomes that would be optimal from either our, or our parasites', perspective. We have a reasonable lead on bacterial intruders; we grossly neglect the protozoan parasites that mainly afflict the third world; we are dangerously ignorant about how to cope with viruses.

Pasteur and Darwin

Charles Darwin's role in nineteenth-century thought, how that shapes our own thinking about man's place in Nature, is too well known and oft discussed to bear extensive elaboration on my part. His contemporary, Louis Pasteur, is a culture hero, world renowned for the human benefits of his germ theory of disease: the use of antiseptic hygiene and of vaccines to prevent infection.

The ideological interaction of these two iconoclasts has been given too little attention. In his correspondence, Darwin makes enthusiastic but passing reference to Pasteur's humanitarian

contributions.[1] Pasteur's correspondence has been less extensively indexed to date.[2] The most notable allusion to Darwin in
his published work is his address to the Sorbonne on April 7,
1864: "Great problems are in question today, which keep all
spirits in suspense: . . . the creation of man several thousand
years or several thousand centuries ago; the fixity of species, . . .
the idea of a useless God." There is little doubt he is referring to
Charles Darwin, whose work had been translated into French in
1862 and promptly aroused a theological storm. Pasteur is de-
termined, however, to remove himself from that debate and
such mysteries. Instead, he insists on addressing only those questions accessible to experiment, namely, the contemporary claims
of spontaneous generation of microbial life. In 1864, his refuta-
tion was in comfortable support of an orthodoxy that would
invoke the Creator for the ultimate origin of life. Indirectly, it
was an argument against a Darwinian evolution of life arising in
"some warm little pond."[3] Pasteur did show that the plethora of
empirical claims of abiogenesis in sterilized broths exposed to air
could all be accounted for by airborne spread of existing germs.
By 1883, he had returned more optimistically to mechanistic
views of abiogenesis if only one could achieve biochemical asym-
metries, perhaps by the use of electromagnetism. Nevertheless,
there is no record that he ever achieved a sympathetic understanding of Darwinian evolutionary theory; and he seems always
to have been hostile to a methodology of inference, like Darwin's, that deviated from the grain of laboratory experiment.[4]

[1] Darwin to Bentham, 1863; Darwin to Romanes, 1875.

[2] Pasteur's correspondence is being opened to scholars at the archives of L'Institut
Pasteur, Paris.

[3] Charles Darwin to J. D. Hooker (1871). "It is often said that all the conditions for
the first production of a living organism are now present, which could ever have been
present. But if (and oh! what a big if!) we could conceive in some warm little pond,
with all sorts of ammonia and phosphoric salts, light, heat, electricity, &c., present, that
a protein compound was chemically formed ready to undergo still more complex
changes, at the present day such matter would be instantly devoured or absorbed,
which would not have been the case before living creatures were formed."

[4] John Farley, "The Social, Political, and Religious Background to the Work of Louis
Pasteur," *Annual Review of Microbiology* 32 (1978): 133–154.

On Darwin's side, for all his appreciation of Pasteur's medical contributions, he seems never to have incorporated microbiology into his natural history. And, as we know, neither of them had any inkling of two other contemporaries' contribution to fundamental biological understanding. Gregor Mendel's foundations of genetics, articulated in 1865, were buried until 1900. Friedrich Miescher had discovered nucleic acids (DNA) in pus cells in 1870; we were not to begin to understand the biological function of DNA until Avery, MacLeod, and McCarty's work at the Rockefeller Institute in 1944.[5] The latency of DNA research may be ascribed mainly to deficiencies in experimental technique whose repair needed decades of drudgery and many instrumental inventions. The barriers among Darwin, Pasteur, and Mendel were purely cerebral and ideological.

What lost opportunity! Darwin might have found, as present-day investigators do, marvelous experimental material for the study of evolution in populations of microbes—where generation time is measured in minutes, and where natural (or artificial) selection can be applied to tens or hundreds of billions of unicellular organisms at small cost and less ethical compunction. Pasteur and his successors in microbiology might have avoided decades of muddled thinking about variation in bacteria. The revolution in biotechnology could have had a couple of decades' head start. I should not complain: I had the fun and advantage in 1946 of exploring a terra still incognita (genetics of bacteria) that might otherwise have been blanketed with homestead claims for four or five prior decades.[6]

Plagues

Darwin had placed *Homo sapiens* at the pinnacle of the

[5] O. T. Avery, C. M. MacLeod, and M. McCarty, "Studies on the Chemical Nature of the Substance Inducing Transformation of Pneumococcal Types," *Journal of Experimental Medicine* 79 (1944): 137–518.

[6] H. A. Zuckerman and J. Lederberg, "Forty Years of Genetic Recombination in Bacteria: Postmature Scientific Discovery?," *Nature* 327 (1986): 629–631.

evolutionary process, but with as much emphasis on pinnacle as on evolution. He never quite rectified the view that man has a privileged place in nature. Man's intelligence, his culture, his technology has of course left all other plant and animal species out of the competition. Darwin was oblivious about microbes as our competitors of last resort. In experimental science, the Darwinian and Pasteurian perspectives are at last fully integrated. The study of mechanisms of virulence is a top priority in research laboratories applying the most advanced techniques of molecular genetics. Since Theobald Smith in 1934, F. M. Burnet and R. Dubos[7] have offered us broad perspectives of the natural history of infectious disease— perspectives that leave no illusions about the feasibility of eradicating our scourges, of the ongoing struggle. For a period, the works of Paul de Kruif dramatized the efforts of the "microbe-hunters."[8] But one legacy of the "miracle drugs," the antibiotics of the 1940s, has been an extraordinary complacency on the part of the broader culture. Most people today are grossly overoptimistic with respect to the means we have available to forfend global epidemics comparable to the Black Death of the fourteenth century (or, on a lesser scale, the influenza of 1918), which took a toll of millions of lives! We have no guarantee that the natural evolutionary competition of viruses with the human species will always find ourselves the winner.

I would ask the professional cultural historians for their comment; but it appears that our half-century has turned away from external nature and to the self-deprecation of human nature, or of human organizations, as the central target of fear and struggle. Not that we have to quarrel over pride of place between virus infection and nuclear doomsday.

---

[7] Theobald Smith, *Parasitism and Disease* (Princeton: Princeton University Press, 1934); F. M. Burnet and D. O. White, *Natural History of Infectious Disease* (Cambridge: Cambridge University Press, 1972); 1st ed. 1940); R. Dubos, *Man Adapting* (New Haven: Yale University Press, 1965). See also Hans Zinsser, *Rats, Lice and History* (Boston: Little Brown, 1935).

[8] Paul de Kruif, *Microbe Hunters* (New York: Harcourt Brace, 1926).

The countercultural protest against technology posits a benign nature, whose balance we now disturb with diabolical modernities. But man himself is a fairly recent emergent on the planet; the sheer growth of our species since the paleolithic is the major source of disturbances to that hypothetical balance. Man as a creature of culture is a man-made species; for better or worse, the only planet we know is a Promethean artifact. Genesis mandates: "Be fruitful and multiply!" After sampling the tree of knowledge, and acquiring the means, we could return to Eden only by reducing the human population to about 1 percent of its current density. We are complacent to trust that nature is benign; we are arrogant to assert that we have the means to except ourselves from the competition. But our principal competitors for dominion, outside our own species, are the microbes: the viruses, bacteria, and parasites. They remain an interminable threat to our survival.

This harsh view may be a product of my day-to-day laboratory experience. Most of my own scientific contributions have entailed the relentless use of artificial selection[9] as a way to detect rare differences in the genetic makeup of individuals in large populations. These were populations of bacteria; but they numbered in the billions in each test tube. Typically, all but a few of these would be wiped out by the chemical or virus intentionally added to remove that "normal background"; a few survivors of uncharacteristic genetic composition are then readily detected and isolated. So I have personally observed, even contrived, the wipeout of populations on a gigascale, and of course recognize that this is an unremitting process in nature—for example, recovery from infection on the part of any patient. This may come about either by the administration of an antibiotic or the mobilization of the naturally evolved defense mechanisms of the patient. In such confrontations, either the human individual or billions of microbes must die.

[9] J. Lederberg, "The Ontogeny of the Clonal Selection Theory of Antibody Formation: Reflections on Charles Darwin and Paul Ehrlich," *Annals N.Y. Acad. Sci.* 546 (1988): 175–187.

As Twort and d'Herelle first observed over seventy years ago, such competition can be seen within the microbial world, in nature or in the microcosms of the test tube: for bacteria have their own viruses, often in uneasy equilibrium with their hosts. It is not unusual to observe a thriving bacterial population of a billion cells undergo a dramatic wipeout, a massive lysis, a sudden clearing of the broth, in consequence of a spontaneous mutation extending the host range of a single virus particle. The bacteria will be succeeded by a hundred billion viruses—whose own fate is now problematical, as they will have exhausted their prey (within that test tube). There may, or may not, sometimes be a few bacterial survivors, mutant bacteria that now resist the mutant virus; if so these can repopulate the test tube—until perhaps a second round, a mutant-mutant virus appears.

Is there any reason to believe that such processes are unique to the test tube, that life in the large is exempt from them? Of course not! Only the time scale is certain to be different, by a factor of years to minutes, of a million to one, the disparity of generation time of human to bacteria. The fundamental biological principles are the same. The numerical odds may be different, by a factor hard to estimate.

As crowded as we are, humans are more dispersed over the planetary surface than are the "bugs" in a glass tube, and we have somewhat fewer opportunities to infect one another, jet airplanes notwithstanding. The culture medium in the test tube offers fewer chemical and physical barriers to virus transmission than the space between people—but you will understand why so many diseases are sexually transmitted. The ozone shield still lets through enough solar ultraviolet light to make aerosol transmission less hospitable; and most viruses are fairly vulnerable to desiccation in dry air. The unbroken skin is an excellent barrier to infection; the mucous membranes of the respiratory tract much less so. And we have evolved immune defenses, a wonderfully intricate machinery for producing a panoply of antibodies, each specifically attuned to the chemical makeup of a particular invading parasite. In the normal, immune-competent individual, each incipient infection is a mortal race: between the penetration and proliferation of the virus within the body, and the development of antibodies that will dampen or extinguish the infection. If we have been vaccinated or infected before with a virus related to the current infection, we can mobilize an early immune response. But this in turn provides selective pressure on the virus populations, encouraging the emergence of antigenic variants. We see this most dramatically in the influenza pandemics; and every few years we need to disseminate fresh vaccines to cope with the current generation of the flu virus.[10]

Many quantitative mitigations of the pandemic viral threat are then inherent in our evolved biological capabilities of coping with these competitors. Mitigation is also built into the evolution of the virus: it is a pyrrhic victory for a virus to eradicate its host! This may have happened historically, but then both that vanquished host and the victorious parasite will have disappeared. Even the death of the single infected individual is relatively disadvantageous, in the long run, to the virus—compared to a sustained infection leaving a carrier free to spread the virus to as many contacts as possible. From the virus's perspective, its ideal would be a virtually symptomless infection, in which the host is quite oblivious of providing shelter and nourishment for the indefinite propagation of the virus's genes. Our own genome probably carries hundreds of thousands of such stowaways. The boundary between them and the "normal genome" is quite blurred; intrinsic to our own ancestry and nature are not only Adam and Eve, but any number of invisible germs that have crept into our chromosomes. Some confer incidental and mutual benefit. Others of these symbiotic viruses (or "plasmids"[11]) have reemerged as oncogenes, with the potential of mutating to a state that we

---

[10] E. D. Kilbourne, *Influenza* (New York: Plenum Medical, 1987).

[11] J. Lederberg, "Cell Genetics and Hereditary Symbiosis," *Physiology Review* 32 (1952): 403–430.

recognize as the dysregulated cell growth of a cancer. As much as 95 percent of our DNA may be "selfish," parasitic in origin.

At evolutionary equilibrium, we would continue to share the planet with our parasites, paying some tribute but deriving some protection from them against more violent aggression. Such an equilibrium is unlikely on terms we would voluntarily welcome: at the margin, the comfort and precariousness of life would be evenly shared. No theory lets us calculate the details; we can hardly be sure that such an equilibrium for earth even includes the human species. Many prophets have foreseen the contrary, given our propensity for technological sophistication harnessed to intraspecies competition.

In fact, innumerable perturbations remind us that we cannot rely on "equilibrium"—each individual death of an infected person is a counterexample. Our defense mechanisms do not always work; viruses are not always as benign as would be predicted to serve their long-term advantage.

The historic plagues, the Black Death of the fourteenth century, the recurrences of cholera, the 1918 swine influenza should be constant reminders of nature's sword over our head. They have been very much on my mind for the past two decades.[12] However, when I have voiced such fears, they have been mollified by the expectation that modern hygiene and medicine would contain any such outbreaks. There is, of course, much merit in those expectations: the plague bacillus is susceptible to antibiotics, and we understand its transmission by rat-borne fleas. Cholera can be treated fairly successfully with simple regimens like oral rehydration (salted water with a touch of sugar). Influenza in 1918 was undoubtedly complicated by bacterial infections that could now be treated with antibiotics; and if we can mobilize them in

[12] J. Lederberg, "Biological Warfare and the Extinction of Man," *Stanford M. D.* 8 (Fall 1969): 15–18; J. Lederberg, "Orthobiosis: The Perfection of Man," in Arne Tiselius and Sam Nilsson, eds., *The Place of Value in a World of Facts: Nobel Symposium XIV* (New York: John Wiley & Sons, 1970); J. Lederberg, "The Infamous Black Death May Return to Haunt Us," *Washington Post,* Aug. 31, 1968.

time, vaccines can help prevent the global spread of a new flu. On the other hand, the role of secondary bacterial infection in 1918 may well be overstated: it is entirely possible that the virus itself was extraordinarily lethal. The retrospective scoffing at the federal campaign against the swine flu of 1976 is a cheap shot on the part of critics who have no burden of responsibility for a wrong guess. It underrates health officials' legitimate anxiety that we might have been seeing a recurrence of 1918[13]—and underscores the political difficulty of undertaking the measures that might be needed in the face of a truly species-threatening pandemic. This so-called fiasco in fact mitigated an epidemic that happily proved to be of a less lethal virus strain. The few cases of side-effects attributed to the (polyvalent) vaccine are undoubtedly less than would have appeared from the flu infections avoided by the vaccination program. However, the incentives to attach fault for damages from a positive intervention have predictable consequences in litigation, not to be confused with the balance of social costs and benefits of the program as a whole.

Many outbreaks of viral or bacterial infections have destroyed large herds of animals, of various species, usually leaving a few immune survivors. With all the discussion of faunal extinctions, nothing has been said about infectious disease. It would be impossible to verify this from the fossil record, but disease is the most plausible mechanism of episodic shifts in populations. Incontrovertible examples of species wipeouts are seen with fungi in the plant world: Dutch elm disease and the American chestnut blight. Yes, it can happen.

My discussion has emphasized viruses because medical science has still to develop effective drugs for the treatment of virus infections—we have but a small handful, of limited use. Keep in mind that bacteria are free-living organisms whose metabolic peculiarities lend themselves to differential attack. For example, the bacterial cell wall is utterly unlike any

[13] Kilbourne, *Influenza.*

structure found in human cells. Hence, penicillin, which attacks the integrity of the bacterial cell wall, is all but innocuous to human tissue, and can be given in very large doses so as to saturate every susceptible bacterial cell. Viruses, on the other hand, are genetic fragments which live within the host cells and exploit their metabolism. It has so far been very difficult to find chemicals that will inhibit a virus without harming the host cell at the same time. Our principal strategy for dealing with viruses is immunization, evoking antibodies that recognize the peculiarities of the virus surface. When a virus, like AIDS, comes along and targets the immune system itself, we are left with dimmer hopes of being able to use that strategy; and we have very few alternatives.

Our main concern about bacterial plagues is for the emergence of antibiotic-resistant strains of familiar threats—for example, chloramphenicol-resistant typhoid. Plasmids are known to travel among bacterial strains and confer antibiotic resistance. Hence selective pressures favoring antibiotic-resistant mutations in the bacteria in cattle's intestines (by our routinely feeding them antibiotics) have ended up making it more difficult to treat human disease with the same drugs. Probably even more important, and more difficult to control, is the inappropriate use of antibiotics for trivial human disease, or often for viral infections which antibiotics cannot control anyhow, with the same result. In effect, any antibiotic will have a limited lifetime of practical use; but we have devised no way of rationing that to be sure it saves the most lives. (On the other hand, it has been surmised that the indiscriminate use of penicillin, by purely incidental effect, is the main cause for the drastic mitigation of syphilis in the United States, most cases having been treated unintentionally. Here we have been unaccountably lucky that penicillin-resistant syphilis just hasn't emerged. We don't know why.) We have been in a well-chronicled race: human wit in the development of new antibiotics versus the evolutionary drive for the emergence of resistant mutants. We gained an enormous lead during the

1940s' discoveries of these magic bullets; on the whole we probably have the appropriate incentives and scientific understanding to retain that lead, at least in the developed countries. As must be reiterated, our neglect of infectious disease in the poor majority of the world is not just a humanitarian disgrace; it leaves unchecked the seeds of our parochial infection.

Besides drug-resistance, bacteria do have some surprises for us: in recent history, the spreading tick-borne epidemic of Lyme arthritis and the storied Legionella show what can emerge overnight; and how perplexing that can be until the parasite is isolated and identified. Other mysterious variations in lethality of bacterial infections come to notice from time to time. Besides the fluctuations of environment that are usually invoked, closer attention should be given to the likelihood that the bacteria themselves may undergo genetic evolution. This may be alarming, insofar as we cannot be sure that the plague bacilli we see today, and believe we can control, are just the same as those responsible for the fourteenth-century pandemic.

Technology's impact is not all on the human side of the struggle. Monoculture of plants and animals has, of course, made them more exposed to devastation. In like fashion, the increasing density of human habitations, inventions like the subway and the jet airplane, all add to the risks of spread of infection. Paradoxically, improvements in sanitation and vaccination leave the larger human herd more innocent of microbial experience, and may in the long run make us the more vulnerable. On the other hand, the loosening of ethnic barriers has made the human population a mite more variable, and in principle better equipped to deal with biological challenges. Evolutionary modes of adaptation, we must never forget, carry a terrible cost in the lives of extant individuals. The best-known example in the human is the sickle cell trait, evolved in Africa as an adaptation to malarial infection. The ancestral benefit to the heterozygotes is exacting a cost today in sickle cell disease among the homozygotes, about two births per thousand among American blacks. The evolutionary calculus tells us this will come to equilibrium only when as many homozygotes have died (or will not be born) as ancestral heterozygotes had been saved from malaria. Infectious disease has undoubtedly loomed large among the selective factors shaping the human genome, and eventually will help explain the polymorphisms in blood groups and in histocompatibility (tissue-graft) antigens. We have had plausible speculations that genetic diseases like the Tay-Sachs syndrome may have conferred some protection against tuberculosis.

Technology, manifest in the opening of wild lands to human occupation, has also exposed people to unaccustomed animal viruses, to zoonoses. Yellow fever has sustained reservoirs in jungle primates, and the same source is the probable origin of the HIV virus in Africa. It is mystifying that yellow fever has not become endemic in India, where competent mosquitoes and susceptible people abound. We will almost certainly be having like experiences from the "opening" of the Amazon basin.

More remote, perhaps more farfetched, is the interplanetary transfer of infection. My own concerns, since Sputnik,[14] have addressed the need to quarantine the planets, more to protect them from contamination from a germ-laden earth than vice versa. The main values at stake are in scientific understanding, which will certainly be confused should we find bacterial spores on Mars and have not undertaken hygienic precautions beforehand. So long as we do not rush people to Mars (which bears the concomitant imperative of returning them to earth), we can do all the necessary preliminary science with clean, unmanned missions, as has been internationally agreed policy to date.

AIDS and Other Plagues

The sudden and tragic spread of AIDS has brought us back

[14] J. Lederberg, "Sputnik 1957–1987," *Scientist*, Oct. 5, 1987.

to earth in our speculation on plagues: who among us has not been personally touched already! A host of social and ethical issues come right to home, and will be the main focus of this conference. As always, the third world is paying the heaviest price, in the dying of whole villages and in the stigma of the biological origins of the virus. We are all in fear of what will come next. Will the virus spread still further? What are the prospects of a vaccine? Of a cure?

You will have professional epidemiologists speak to the current statistics. There is nothing hopeful about them. But you should not think that AIDS is our only plague. In the third world, tuberculosis and malaria are until now just as devastating in their public-health impact, and are likely to remain deathly competitors to AIDS in toll on human life. Unlike AIDS, most of the third world endemics are most painful as chronic diseases, which kill millions to be sure but leave many more in debilitation and suffering, still-hungry mouths to be fed. On top of those, over 3 million children a year die of diarrheal disease, a like number from infections for which effective vaccines exist but have not been available where needed. This enormous mortality is entirely preventable. The neglect of it is related to the history of a new disease that must have been spreading unremarked in Africa for ten or fifteen years before it emerged in the Western Hemisphere. Nor will AIDS be the last example of its kind.

We are all too familiar with the factors that have made AIDS an especially ugly challenge. Unlike other virus infections, which leave some survivors immune to further attack, there is nothing in the natural history of AIDS to point either to a cure or to a vaccine. Victims develop antibodies, then go on notwithstanding to develop more aggravated disease, with the eventual collapse of the immune system. The fact that this is still mysterious makes it the most promising avenue for new discovery and possible intervention. Most of the factual knowledge we have is unremittingly discouraging.

The long latent period multiplies the opportunity for

spread; the victim may be unaware of carrying the virus, even less his contacts. Nothing could provoke more anxiety than this protracted uncertainty. The targeting of the immune system also encourages the seeding of other infections—we are already starting to see a recrudescence of tuberculosis in the United States and aggravations of syphilis and a host of opportunistic organisms rarely seen before. It would be far worse were HIV still more readily spread, but its substantial confinement to special high-risk groups worsens the social tensions around efforts at control. The long latent period guarantees a large number of momentarily healthy carriers whose civil rights—for example, to continued schooling and employment—are in instant conflict with a quarantine mentality for public-health control. I was labeled an alarmist twenty years ago for raising a "specter" of pandemic. My most pessimistic imagination did not fetch the constellation of attributes that we observe with AIDS. AIDS is already so prevalent in the United States today that none of the approaches of public-health control of other acute infections are pertinent. There is little merit in targeting a handful of individuals, generally the most compliant, when there are a score as many freely walking the streets.

So much is unknown about AIDS that a large amount of testing is essential just to understand the scope and localization of the problem. We may soon find that many hospital and medical procedures aggravate AIDS infection: that will obligate broader testing of AIDS among hospital admissions, simply for the patients' benefit. And they will sue for not having been routinely tested. Health-care personnel have an ethical obligation to care for all the sick; but this is complemented by a right to know what they need to protect their own health. We will not work out the most viable balance between individual rights and the community's needs without a great deal more compassionate thought and inevitable political stress. Both need to be informed by more reliable knowledge.

Will AIDS get even worse? It may already be worse than we

believe—there is a fair possibility that some potential carriers
are still uncounted, that they will have a long latent period
after primary infection, before the virus reemerges and before
antibodies begin to appear. Such a stage at least is not fraught
with transmitting the disease to others. We have yet to learn
more precisely how readily it can be transmitted by heterosexual contact; there is not much point trying to predict the future
course of AIDS prevalence by simple arithmetic extrapolation,
when utterly different communities and vehicles are involved.
We have Africa as a dismal historic example of progressively
broad spread; and I am not much impressed by arguments
that speak to cultural idiosyncrasies (as opposed to mere time)
as the difference between their experience and ours. Regardless, with what we know we have on our hands, we have a
rough road ahead.

As with some health-care workers, we are likely to
experience a few cases of AIDS transmitted outside the
"high-risk behaviors." As such, these will have a political
impact far beyond their public-health importance, in contrast
to the recognized, dominant modes of transmission. We have
to be careful not to be stampeded by a few tragic accidents
statistically equivalent to lightning bolts. Rarely in human
history has so much rested on the clarity of social decision-
making, subject to extraordinary constraints of group interest,
prejudice, and ignorance.

Will AIDS mutate further? Already known, a vexing feature
of AIDS is its antigenic variability, further complicating the
task of developing a vaccine. So we know that HIV is still
evolving. Its global spread has meant there is far more HIV on
earth today than ever before in history. What are the odds of
its learning the tricks of airborne transmission? The short
answer is, "No one can be sure." But we could make the same
attribution about any virus; alternatively the next influenza or
chicken pox may mutate to an unprecedented lethality. As
time passes, and HIV seems settled in a certain groove, that is
momentary reassurance in itself. However, given its other ugly

attributes, it is hard to imagine a worse threat to humanity than an airborne variant of AIDS. No rule of nature contradicts such a possibility; the proliferation of AIDS cases with secondary pneumonia multiplies the odds of such a mutant, as an analogue to the emergence of pneumonic plague. Such cases warrant and receive close-isolation precautions; but who will ensure that in Africa? We must particularly look more deeply into the biological mechanisms that govern how AIDS can or cannot be transmitted; our current assessments are crude empiricisms. And with so much at stake we must multiply our vigilance for evidence of extraordinary channels of spread.

Our preoccupation with AIDS should not obscure the multiplicity of infectious diseases that threaten our future. It is none too soon to start a systematic watch for other new viruses before they become so irrevocably lodged. The fundamental bases of virus research can hardly be given too much encouragement—and they have made extraordinary leaps, particularly with the help of recombinant DNA technology.[15] Such research should be done on a broad international scale, both to share the progress made in advanced countries and to amplify the opportunities for fieldwork in the most afflicted ones.

We also have some political lessons learned. Hard-won human rights, the autonomy of individuals, will be in conflict with the quietude of the community. At severe cost, if at all, will it be possible to impose traditional disease-control methods like isolation and quarantine on new viruses. Compulsory

[15] The sensational publicity given ca. 1975 to the hypothetical hazards of recombinant DNA research ignited public fears and regulatory reactions that boded ill for the opportunity to continue research on methodology of the most crucial importance for the understanding of virus infection. Some participants at the much-heralded Asilomar Conference treated such research as if it were an idle diversion for the amusement of scientists; therefore what harm in an indefinite moratorium? See J. Lederberg, "DNA Research: Uncertain Peril and Certain Promise," in J.D. Watson and J. Tooze, *The DNA Story: A Documentary History of Gene Cloning* (San Francisco: Freeman, 1981).

vaccination has all but passed the pale. Claims for redress for individual harm from medical accidents from vaccines necessitate that we find new social-insurance approaches to indemnification. Failing that, we have already seen a collapse of the pharmaceutical industry's incentive and capability for pursuing new vaccine developments. The most stunning victories will be quiet ones, against viruses we have learned enough about beforehand to keep them from planting a foothold.

The stresses on democratic civility posed by AIDS have no precedent in U.S. history. They are compounded by our scientific uncertainties as to where this epidemic is heading. The best available advice is incorporated in the program advocated by the leadership of the federal health agencies and the expertise of groups like the National Academy of Sciences.[16] That advice can be no more authentic than the empirical findings to date. It is of the greatest urgency that these be bolstered by a more robust appreciation of virus biology and of the human immune mechanism. At present, nothing we know gives us assurance of finding satisfactory cures or vaccines for AIDS infection. We can take small comfort that much more remains to be explored—but only if we mount that exploration with the most urgent priority.

Additional Comments

P. 28. The general theme that virus-host relationships evolve towards less virulent, stable commensalism has been criticized by R. M. May and R. M. Anderson. "Parasite—host coevolution." *Parasitology* 100: S89–S101, 1990. They stress that selection within the infected host favors the more virulent geno-

---

[16] Institute of Medicine, National Academy of Sciences, *Confronting AIDS: Directions for Public Health, Health Care, and Research* (Washington, 1986). Regarding AIDS see more recently: Eve K. Nichols, *Mobilizing Against AIDS* (Washington: National Academy of Sciences, 1989); H. Mitsuya, R. Yarchoan, and S. Broder, "Molecular Targets for AIDS Therapy," *Science* 249 (1990): 1533–1544; A. S. Fauci, "The Human Immunodeficiency Virus—Infectivity and Mechanisms of Pathogenesis," *Science* 239 (1988): 617–622; Hung Fan et al., *The Biology of AIDS* (Boston: Jones & Bartlett, 1989).

types, however this may result in a deprivation of prey for further spread of the parasite. Nevertheless, many stable commensalisms and mutualistic symbioses have indeed evolved, culminating in the incorporation of mitochondria and chloroplasts as essential constituents of animal and plant cells. Cf. L. Margulis, *Symbiosis in Cell Evolution.* San Francisco: Freeman, 1982.

P. 32. For further detail on looming threats from new and emerging viruses, see Stephen Morse, ed., *Emerging Viruses.* Princeton: Princeton University Press, to be published in 1991.

P. 35. Three years' further experience has fortunately given no direct evidence of more facile spread of HIV, e.g., by airborne transmission. We have only the general comfort that HIV "is not very infectious" as theoretical grounding for this observation, and continued vigilance remains warranted. Antigenic variability of HIV does appear to be a complication for efforts to develop a vaccine. T. F. W. Wolfs, et al. "Evolution of Sequences Encoding the Principal Neutralization Epitope of Human Immuno-deficiency Virus 1 Is Host Dependent, Rapid, and Continuous." *Proc. Nat. Acad. Sci. U.S.* 87 (1990): 9938–9942.

Addendum to Footnotes

1. C. Darwin to G. Bentham, May 22, 1863. Darwin to F. Holmgren, April 14, 1881. Darwin to F. J. Cohn, January 3, 1878: The calendar to Darwin's correspondence, on the other hand, records several letters from medical people inquiring about the correlation of evolutionary principles to infection, but with no reply indicated. See F. Burkhardt and S. Smith, eds., *A Calendar of the Correspondence of Charles Darwin, 1821–1882. (New York: Garland, 1985).*

3. *The calendar (v.s.{1}) remarks that Pasteur's experiment on abiogenesis is mentioned in this letter, which has not been published in full text to date.*

Placing Blame for Devastating Disease

BY DOROTHY NELKIN
AND SANDER L. GILMAN

IN October 1985 a long article entitled "Panic in the West: or, What Hides Behind the Sensationalism of AIDS" appeared in *Literaturnaya Gazeta*, the official journal of the Soviet Writers Union. Shortly thereafter the journal printed a detailed interview on the same topic with Professor S. Drozdov, the director of the Research Institute of Poliomyelitis and Encephalitis in Moscow.[1] The theme of both articles was the same—AIDS was the result of a virus, man-made by the biological warriors at Fort Detrick, Maryland, in conjunction with the scientists at the Centers for Disease Control in Atlanta, Georgia. That blame for this dread disease was placed on a political adversary is not very surprising in light of the freeze on American-Soviet relations during the summer of 1985. More fascinating are the associations evoked by the political cartoonist for *Pravda*, D. Agaeva. His cartoon represents an American general paying for a test tube of AIDS virus supplied to him by a venal-looking scientist. Swimming about in the test tube, representing the power of the AIDS virus, are a multitude of tiny swastikas; the dead, the victims of AIDS, appear in the cartoon as concentration-camp victims, their bare feet echoing the death-camp photographs of bodies stacked like cordwood with only their feet showing.

Placing the blame for AIDS on America worked only until

---

[1] See J. Seale, "AIDS Virus Infection: A Soviet View of Its Origin," *Journal of the Royal Society of Medicine* 79 (1986): 494–495.

the Soviets, in the climate of *glasnost* in late 1986, admitted that
they too had indigenous cases of the disease. But during 1985
and early 1986 the Soviet press was projecting an image of the
United States as fascist and degenerate. Some Russians viewed
homosexuality as a pathological reflex of late forms of
capitalism and AIDS as a reflection of Western government
and society. Thus, in one powerful image, the *Pravda*
cartoonist managed to draw an association between American
imperialism, Nazi fascism, and dread disease.

The placing of blame has been a pervasive theme in the
popular discourse on AIDS. Since 1981, when the first case of
AIDS was identified, blame for the disease has been placed
variously on dangerous lifestyles, on immoral behavior, on
intravenous drug use, on "poppers," on the CIA, on dioxin
and Agent Orange, on government policies, on Haitians (by
the American media), or on Americans (by the French).

Blaming has always been a means to make mysterious and
devastating diseases comprehensible and therefore possibly
controllable. Even when disease was routinely assumed to be
caused by "God's will," "the Lord's wrath," or "occult
influences," people looked for the behavior that was to blame
for divine judgment and retribution. It is commonly assumed
that modern scientific understanding of infection and contagion has neutralized such folkloric views of disease, that the
political and moral judgments that were so characteristic of
premodern societies are relics of the past. But diseases are
never fully understood. And so we still make moral judgments
for misfortune. We still point the finger of blame.[2] In a
situation of communal anxiety, locating blame for disease is in
effect a strategy of control. If responsibility can be fixed,
perhaps something—discipline, prudence, isolation—can be
done.

Locating blame is in effect a quest for order and certainty in

[2] This argument extends to the popular discourse on risk. See Mary Douglas and
Aaron Wildavsky, *Risk and Culture* (Berkeley: University of California Press, 1982).

an anxious and disruptive situation. It is a particularly pervasive syndrome when science and medicine are perceived as impotent. Thus the rhetoric of blame is most evident today in the discourse on the causes of diseases such as AIDS or cancer, while historically it appeared in discussions of leprosy, syphilis, or plague. These are situations where medical science has failed to serve as a source of definitive understanding and control, so people try to create their own order and to reduce their own sense of vulnerability. In effect, placing blame defines the normal, establishes the boundaries of healthy behavior and appropriate social relationships, and distinguishes the observer from the cause of fear.

Categories of blame often reflect deep social-class biases. Illness is frequently associated with poverty and becomes a justification for social inequities. But blaming is also a way to create psychological as well as social boundaries. For the individual, blame is a way to draw a boundary between the self and the diseased, and thereby to release anxiety. To make stereotypical definitions of who is at risk is, of course, to fantasize. But disease is frequently associated with the "other," be it the other race, the other class, the other ethnic group.[3] Inevitably the locus of blame is also tied to specific ideological, political, and social concerns. Blame is in effect a social construct, a reflection of the worldviews, social stereotypes, and political biases that prevail at a given time.[4]

In this context, we will explore some patterns in the location of blame for disease as they have appeared in the popular writing and media reports on catastrophic and contagious disease throughout history. Several categories of blame can be found in this popular discourse: disease has been attributed to particular racial groups or social stereotypes, to individual lifestyle, to immoral behavior, or to those perceived as sources of power and control.

---

[3] This is carefully documented in the case of venereal disease by Allan Brandt, *No Magic Bullet,* 2nd ed. (New York: Oxford University Press, 1987).

[4] Mary Douglas, *Purity and Danger* (London: Penguin, 1970).

Racial Groups or Social Stereotypes

In the early 1980s public-health officials considered Haitians to be one of the major sources of AIDS in the United States. Whatever the origin of AIDS, and this is not at all clear, it was very quickly labeled an African or Haitian disease. Ironically, however, the French in 1981 labeled AIDS an American disease, observing the influence of American cultural models of homosexuality in France. For some, AIDS was but another example of the American corruption of the French body politic, but now in the form of a "real" disease. Jacques Liebowitz, a physician working in Paris, reported the prevailing belief that AIDS was caused by the importation from the United States of contaminated "poppers" (amyl nitrate), a chemical used to heighten sexual experiences and strongly associated with the homosexual lifestyle. The French press had described poppers as "an American pollutant consumed here." And the French government then warned the Franco-American gay jet set that they were at risk because of their "American connection."[5]

The location of blame "over there" was a characteristic aspect of the myths that developed over many centuries to explain syphilis. For sixteenth-century writers, syphilis *had* to come from the New World: it was the final sign of the cataclysmic changes of that period, from the creation of the middle class to the reappearance of the Black Death. It signified the disruption of the old order and the dissolution of the hierarchies of the Old World. Syphilis terrified the Europeans during the first decades after the discovery of the New World. As it became necessary to distinguish the goals of European colonialism from those of the indigenous population, Indians became not only diseased, they were defined as the source of the disease. The very image of the Indian

[5] Jacques Liebowitz, *A Strange Virus of Unknown Origin* (New York: Ballantine, 1985), p. 5.

changed. In the illustrated reports of the first explorers they were portrayed as the classic Greek, clothed in a toga. Later they were perceived as the polluted primitive; the healthy became the dangerous and diseased.[6] Yet when the Indians of the New World were being relentlessly destroyed in the colonial mines, Las Casas, a priest, wrote to the king of Spain, observing that the real "disease" which had to be cured was not syphilis but Spanish colonialism. This, he claimed, was killing the Indians more certainly than syphilis was destroying the Europeans.[7]

The increased movement of people across national borders reinforced the need to protect social boundaries. Every national group in Europe defined syphilis as a disease of other nations. A 1524 tract on syphilis listed over 200 names for the disease, each identifying it as originating in a specific location.[8] For the Germans it was the French disease, for the French the Italian disease. Fracastor's famous work on syphilis in the sixteenth century called it *Morbus Gallicus,* the French disease.[9] Erasmus, a Dutchman, associated syphilis with German inns. He described the crude manners, the excessive and immoral social interaction in German as contrasted to French inns. "Quite apart from the belching of garlic, the breaking of wind, the stinking breaths, many person suffer from hidden diseases, and every disease is contagious."[10] An eighteenth-century study of venereal disease added that the Japanese called it the disease of the Portuguese, the Persians called it a disease of the Turks, and the Poles the disease of the Russians.[11] By the late

[6] Benedet Bucher, *La Sauvage aux Siens Pendant* (Paris: Hermann, 1977).

[7] Bartolomé de Las Casas, *Historia de las Indias* (Madrid: M. Ginesta, 1975–76), p. 192. See also discussion in Theodore Rosebury, *Microbes and Morals* (New York: Ballantine Books, 1973).

[8] Ulrich von Hutten, in Henrach Apenheimer, ed., *Uber die Hilkarft des Guaraium* (Berlin: August Hirschwald, 1902).

[9] Fracastor, "Syphilis sive Morbus Gallicus," 1530.

[10] Orban Goudsblom, "Public Health and the Civilizing Process," *Milbank Quarterly* 641 (1986): 171.

[11] J. A. Astruc, *A Treatise of Venereal Disease* (London: Innis, Richardson, Davis & Cox, 1754).

nineteenth century a different theory of syphilis appears in popular discourse. It was not a disease introduced into Europe by Columbus's sailors, but rather a form of leprosy long present in Africa, brought to Europe by blacks during the Middle Ages.[12]

The poor have frequently been set apart by identifying them with disease. In his classic book, *How the Other Half Lives,* the reporter and social-reform advocate Jacob Riis dwells on the diseases of the poor in "Jewtown": "Typhus fever and smallpox are bred here. . . . Filthy diseases both, they sprout naturally among the hoards that bring the germs with them from across the sea." In this slum where ready-made clothes were made in tenements, Riis imagines a smallpox or typhus fever patient in a room where bundles of coats are made to be sold to the public in department stores, "each one lined with the wearer's death warrant, unseen and unsuspected, basted in the lining."[13]

The "smell" of the poor has frequently been cited as evidence of disease.[14] Just as physicians in the Middle Ages claimed that Jews emitted the *foetor judaicus,* the sulfuric smell believed to be the cause of illness and death, so too the poor were believed to stink. The British in the 1840s saw cholera as the result of the "effluvia" present in those crowded, squalid neighborhoods populated by the poor and working class. Soho, a poor neighborhood in the center of London, was the center of the 1848–49 outbreak of cholera. The official explanation for this was the disgusting smell that was ever-present on Soho's streets. Given the crazy-quilt pattern of nineteenth-century London, with well-to-do neighborhoods interspersed by pockets of the direst poverty, people were inclined to relate the spread of cholera to their general fear of the poor. The physician John Snow rejected this thesis and

---

[12] Iwan Bloch, *Der Ursprung der Syphilis,* 2 vols. (Jena: Gustav Fischer, 1901–11).

[13] Jacob A. Riis, *How the Other Half Lives* (Cambridge: Harvard University Press, 1970), p. 73.

[14] Goudsblom, "Public Health."

claimed that the disease was contagious and borne by water, not effluvia. But his view was not given credence until he was able to show definitively that it was not the poverty (and therefore the smell) of a neighborhood that was to blame for the outbreak of cholera but distance from the ever-polluting, but classless, Thames.[15]

Clinical categories, then, are frequently associated with specific groups—sometimes identified by race, sometimes by nationality or social class. In each case, blame for disease turns into a crusade against those who are feared or who, by being different, are viewed as a threat to the established social order.

Immorality

While marginal social groups often carry the burden of blame, explanations of disease often become a means to define appropriate and moral behavior. From its first diagnosis in 1981, most professional reports and the popular press have labeled AIDS, not as a viral disease like hepatitis, but as a sexually transmitted disease like syphilis. The label, of course, stigmatizes those with AIDS and implies that all sexual contact is promiscuous, immoral, and dangerous. Moral judgments are most explicit among right-wing religious groups, who explicitly view AIDS as God's punishment for deviant sexual behavior. But even children with AIDS have been morally stigmatized. Recall the public hearing in Queens, New York, over whether to allow a seven-year-old child diagnosed as having AIDS into the public school. Children who are ill are usually innocents in our pantheon of images of disease, but this child inherited the unclean image of the patient with a sexually transmitted disease. Though the seven-year-old was presumably infected

[15] John Snow, *On the Mode of Communication of Cholera*, 2nd ed. (London: Churchill, 1855). Also see Norman Longmate, *King Cholera: Biography of a Disease* (London: Hamish, 1966).

through a transfusion, a prominent theme in this hearing was the association of AIDS with morally demeaning behavior.[16] The child emerged as somehow impure, polluted, as well as physically impaired. A similar message is conveyed by a (probably) subconscious printing error in the caption of a newspaper photograph of Ryan White, the twelve-year-old child with AIDS who was the focus of a school dispute in Kokomo, Indiana. The caption described Ryan as a "homophiliac [sic] who contracted AIDS through a blood transfusion."[17]

The location of blame for disease in immorality reflects the old religious tradition of using sexual taboos to draw the line between insiders and outsiders, the "pure" and the "polluted," the coreligionists and the sources of pollution. Disease is a means to reinforce sexual mores. It serves as a public sign of the violation of socially defined boundaries. The sick man becomes a sinner; pestilence is the punishment unleashed by divine retribution; disease is the means to cleanse the sin.

The use of disease to define sexual mores was explicit in the discourse on masturbation in the seventeenth and early eighteenth centuries, when it was strongly proscribed by European Protestantism. A medical text called *Onania, or the Horrible Sin of Self-Pollution,* circulated in the 1730s, catalogued the physical destruction caused by masturbation.[18] In a tone more suitable for the pulpit than for a medical monograph, the book attributed everything to masturbation—from baldness to madness to a long, slow, agonizing death. As a violation of a religious and moral taboo, masturbation, it claimed, leads directly to disease.

From its first appearance in 1495, syphilis was associated with debauched sexuality. Though the commercially manufactured

---

[16] Dorothy Nelkin and Stephen Hilgartner, "Disputed Dimensions of Risk: The AIDS Schoolboard Controversy," *Milbank Quarterly* 64 (1986): 118–142.

[17] *Ithaca Journal,* May 1, 1986.

[18] Sander Gilman, *Difference and Pathology* (Ithaca: Cornell University Press, 1985), pp. 191–192.

rubber condom became available in the nineteenth century as a practical means of combating syphilis, the Roman Catholic church strongly opposed its use. In 1826 Leo XII banned the condom because it prevented debauched individuals from suffering a disease that was their necessary and certain punishment for deviating from sacred practices. As Allan Brandt has documented, venereal disease continued well into the twentieth century to be a symbol for a society characterized by corrupt sexuality and moral contamination.[19]

Once associated with syphilis, smallpox inherited its moral stigma. The name itself, *la petite verole,* was derived from the French term for syphilis: *la grosse verole.* The moral stigma attached to smallpox contributed to disputes over inoculation in the eighteenth century, as colonists argued that it was wrong to avoid a disease that was God's punishment for sin. An epidemic was "an affliction pronounced upon the sins of the community."[20] Inoculation, it was believed, could overturn the covenant between God and the community and encourage immoral behavior, as people would no longer be convinced that their suffering resulted from their sins. By the nineteenth century smallpox and syphilis were medically distinguished, but the conceptual connection persisted. As late as the 1920s opponents of smallpox vaccination called it the "syphilization of society."[21]

American public-health reformers of the nineteenth century also drew connections between morality, religion, and disease. John H. Griscom, the principal health officer in New York City in the 1840s, equated health with piety: "The coincidence, or parallelism, of moral degradation and physical disease is plainly apparent to the experienced observer." Griscom placed

---

[19] Brandt, *No Magic Bullet.*

[20] Perry Miller, *The New England Mind from Colony to Province* (Cambridge: Harvard University Press, 1953), p. 349.

[21] Joshua Schwartz, "Small Pox Immunization: Controversial Episodes," in D. Nelkin, ed., *Controversy: The Politics of Technical Decisions* (Beverly Hills: Sage, 1984), p. 208.

the blame for disease on man's own actions, equating cleanliness with godliness: "If we reflect that cleanliness cannot exist without ventilation we must look upon the latter as not only a moral but a religious duty."[22]

Similarly, in 1891 Dr. John Shaw Billings, surgeon general of the United States, observed the epidemiological fact that the death rate of particular wards varied with the poverty of their inhabitants. He concluded that disease was a reflection of the moral failing of "a distinct class of people who are structurally and almost necessarily idle, ignorant, intemperate and more or less vicious, who are failures or the descendants of failures."[23]

Even as biological explanations for disease became widely accepted, the medical and biological sciences were creating clinical categories such as "degeneration" that incorporated social concepts of blame. In a remarkable and influential series of books on public-health reforms, the German physician Edward Reich defined the basic health problem of the late nineteenth century as "degeneration" caused by sexual activity. Deviant behavior demanded the intervention of the state before the entire society succumbed to disease and degeneration.[24]

Individual Lifestyle

In the twentieth century concepts of morality are frequently translated into questions of lifestyle. Looking to lifestyle as the cause of AIDS, the popular press emphasizes that persons with

[22] Quoted in Charles Rosenberg, *No Other Gods* (Baltimore: Johns Hopkins Press, 1976), pp. 112–114. See also Rosenberg's *The Cholera Years* (Chicago: University of Chicago Press, 1962) for discussion of beliefs about the relationship of disease to concepts of sin.

[23] John S. Billings, "Public Health and Municipal Government," *Annals of the American Academy of Political and Social Science* (supplement), February 1891, p. 6.

[24] Edward Reich's books from 1864 to 1868 are summarized in Gilman, *Difference and Pathology*, pp. 196–198, and in Edward Chamberlin and Sander Gilman, eds., *Degeneration: The Dark Side of Progress* (New York: Columbia University Press, 1985).

AIDS are afflicted as a direct result of their chosen lifestyle—their sexual practices or their use of drugs. Blame for the disease is placed, not on a retrovirus, but on its victims, on those who maintain a self-indulgent pattern of behavior that places them at risk. While AIDS is clearly spread through sexual transmission and intravenous drugs, the rhetoric of blame discounts the fact that behavior may not be entirely voluntary. Furthermore, blaming the individual for illness limits the responsibility of the larger society.

In the contemporary American context, the rhetoric of blame has been most evident in the discourse on preventive medicine and its emphasis on individual responsibility. In 1979, a surgeon general's report called *Healthy People* concluded that the foremost causes of illness lie in individual behavior.[25] Hailed in the press as the manifesto of a public-health revolution, the report urged extensive changes in lifestyle as the way to avoid disease. Subsequently a series of government reports on chronic diseases has attributed disease to problematic individual behavior: to smoking, dietary habits, or personal excess. John Knowles, former president of the Rockefeller Foundation, framed the issue of health in succinct terms by quoting Pogo: "We have met the enemy and he is us."[26]

This tendency to place blame on individual behavior is a ubiquitous theme in the press coverage of many chronic and poorly understood diseases. In the last few years the popular rhetoric on the sources of cancer has focused on the individual's failure to minimize "risk factors," in particular, on reluctance to change eating habits. "Every time you go for that extra pat of butter just think, 'What if I become one of the 38,400 breast cancer fatalities this year?' " "Americans are too

[25] Surgeon General, *Healthy People: The Surgeon General's Report on Health Promotion and Disease Prevention* (Washington: U.S. Department of Health, Education and Welfare, 1979).
[26] John Knowles, "Responsibility for Health," *Science* 198 (December 1977): 1103.

locked into their eggs and bacon."[27] The Puritan lifestyle has become an ideal, and food has become, in effect, a preventive medicine.

While the rhetoric reflects some reality—smoking does cause cancer—such popular explanations often reflect social factors that extend well beyond the results of scientific research on the etiology of disease. There is considerable public frustration with the slow progress in realizing the therapeutic interventions promised by the "war on cancer." And in a conservative political climate there is also political reluctance to associate cancer with exposure to industrial pollutants or occupational carcinogens. Attributing cancer to lifestyle has popular appeal because it appears to enhance individual control over the disease without threatening social or political institutions. A spokesperson for the American Institute for Cancer Research claims that people are "hungry for information" about the effect of lifestyle as a cause of cancer. Explanations such as genetics, viruses, or industrial pollution seem to leave our lives "in the hands of outside forces over which we have little or no say. . . . People see in diet and nutrition the chance to hold in their own hands some measure of control regarding this terrible disease."[28]

Despite scientific evidence to the contrary, diabetes has also been blamed on individual behavior. A popular self-help book on diabetes by Robert Cantu blames adult-onset diabetes on overweight and lack of exercise. He suggests that 90 percent of adult-onset diabetes is preventable with the proper dietary exercise regime. He goes on to express a moral judgment: "If this is true, why is diabetes increasing? One reason is that many people are careless and lazy about their health."[29] Again,

---

[27] These and similar quotes can be found in popular magazines and especially in *Prevention*, which is entirely focused on lifestyle as a cause of disease.

[28] Susan Pepper, speech at the American Institute for Cancer Research, Diet and Cancer Symposium, Washington, D.C., September 1986.

[29] Robert C. Cantu, *Diabetes and Exercise* (New York: E. P. Dutton, 1982). His theories were extensively reported in *Prevention* magazine.

responsibility is placed on individual lifestyle, suggesting that illness is a matter of choice and can be controlled by changes in behavior.

Perhaps the most common explanation of inexplicable diseases these days is "stress," a popular euphemism based on the association of illness with lifestyle. The first question in a survey put out by the American Cancer Research Fund is "Were you aware that experts report as much as 70% of illness, including cancer, may be caused by stress?" Attributing disease to stress is not new. In the late nineteenth century popular and professional writing defined "neurasthenia," or "lack of nerve force," as the primary mental and physical disability of modern society.[30] It was believed to originate in the stress resulting from the increased speed of daily life. For Europeans, and for those Americans, such as Henry Adams, who questioned the implications of technological change, speed was typified by the steam engine, which, despite its origin, became identified with the American way of life. George M. Beard, in his book *American Nervousness,* believed the technologies of modern civilization were to blame for nervousness. The Berlin psychiatrist P.J. Moebius wrote: "It has been correctly observed that the use of steam is the signature of our time. Indeed the introduction of the steam engine has made the steam increase the tempo of modern life; we live with steam."[31]

In the Victorian age, specific categories of individuals were perceived to be at risk from this life in the fast, steam-driven lane. For the Europeans it was the Americans who epitomized this stressful lifestyle. But these "Americans" did not merely live in the United States. In Vienna a local group was also stigmatized as the "Americans among us." According to Richard Krafft-Ebing, Jews in Vienna at the turn of the

---

[30] Gilman, *Difference and Pathology,* p. 156.

[31] George M. Beard, *American Nervousness: Its Cause and Consequences* (New York: G. P. Putnam, 1881), Preface; P. J. Moebius, *Die Nervosität* (Leipzig: J. J. Weber, 1982), p. 87. See also George Frederick Drinka, *The Birth of Neurosis* (New York: Simon & Schuster, 1984), ch. 5, "The Railway God."

century were especially vulnerable to mental illness because they were "overachievers[s] in the arena of commerce or politics," for whom "time is money." They "read reports, business correspondence, [and] stock market notations during meals."[32]

Such lifestyle explanations of disease are particularly subject to prevailing cultural biases. Some diseases brought on by individual behavior are associated with upper-class and status-filled social positions. Gout is a condition that almost assigns social position to its victims. Similarly, stress-related illness among executives is a sign of social mobility. Among others, however, the same disease may be defined in negative terms as a product of deviant or excessive behavior. As the outsiders in Vienna, Jews were stigmatized by stress as "overachievers" involved in the activity—immoral in a class-bound culture—of getting rich.

Sources of Power

A provocative poster, pasted conspicuously on mailboxes throughout Manhattan, is headlined "AIDS is Germ Warfare by U.S. Government." Printed by the United Front Against Racism and Capitalist Imperialism, the poster blames AIDS on the CIA, which it claims has conducted "AIDS bio-warfare directed mainly against gays." The argument spelled out in the poster is that the CIA, acting on behalf of "capitalist ruling circles," is scapegoating blacks and homosexuals, and using AIDS as a scare tactic to mobilize the U.S. masses for right-wing causes. The language is powerful and accusatory, referring to "the false philosophy of eugenics" and "the depraved morality of government." But it is also written in the

---

[32] Richard Krafft-Ebing, *Nervosität und Neurasthenische Zustönde* (Vienna: Hölder, 1895), p. 96.

rhetorical context of the 1980s, using scientific explanations to prove that AIDS is a form of biological warfare.

In 1985 a group of Vietnam veterans began a long lobbying effort to convince the U.S. Congress to investigate their claim that dioxin and Agent Orange are responsible for AIDS. Their literature blames government authorities, the Defense Department, and industrial polluters for causing the disease.[33]

It is perhaps obvious that groups who feel politically marginal should place blame for disease at the feet of government, public officials, or corporate sources of power. Industrial workers, for example, have long placed the blame for tuberculosis and other job-related illnesses on class exploitation. For nonelite groups, disease is a symbol of their resentment of power.

However, placing blame is also a tool in political and professional disputes over power and authority. This was the case in the early eighteenth-century controversy over Dr. Lawrence Dal'honde, a French physician, who testified at public hearings in Boston in 1721 on the merits and dangers of inoculation. His claim that inoculation had caused disease in Europe contributed to the growing public opposition in America and convinced Boston selectmen to ban the smallpox inoculation program.[34] The inoculation dispute during this period reflected competing claims of expertise. The Reverend Cotton Mather, the well-known Calvinist theologian, was the main advocate of inoculation; Dr. William Douglas, the only Boston physician with an M.D. degree, opposed it. Placing blame for the disease on inoculation policies was a means to challenge the intrusion of the clergy into the domain of medical practice.

Blaming responsible authorities for disease has also been a way to express dissatisfaction with unpopular political deci-

---

[33] Reports and correspondence with government and public-health officials and congressional representatives, circulated by Dave Bergh of the Vietnam Support Group in St. Cloud, Minnesota in 1985 and 1986.

[34] Schwartz, "Small Pox Immunization," p. 200.

sions. Witness the polemical discourse about slavery and mental illness in the mid-nineteenth century. The census of 1840 had grossly misreported the number of mentally ill blacks in northern cities, indicating, for example, that in some towns well over half of them were mentally ill. Southern politicians (such as John C. Calhoun), as well as the southern medical establishment, jumped on these "facts" and concluded that mental illness was caused by the inability of blacks to cope with the freedom granted them in the nonslaveholding states. "The negroes, having been suddenly liberated . . . have been freed their customary restraint and fostering care of their former masters," wrote a physician in a southern medical journal.[35] A doctor in New Orleans even coined a new disease entity to explain mental illness among blacks: the "psychosis of freedom." Critics blamed the government and its policies of liberating slaves for creating this "disease."

Conclusion

Perplexing medical questions have always generated fear, prejudice, and hostility. Thus any disease that is poorly understood is freighted with social meaning. The patterns of blame that prevail in different periods reflect the social stereotypes, fears, and political biases that are associated with threats of social or political change. Defining the causes of disease becomes a way to protect existing social categories or power relationships, to define the boundaries of "normal" behavior, or to reinforce the norms that seem to be threatened by marginal groups. By placing blame people seek to create order, to reassert control over perceived threats, or to preserve existing social institutions.

[35] J. C. Nott, "Smallpox Epidemic in Mobile during the Winter of 1865–66," *Nashville Journal of Medical Surgery* 2 (1867): 372–380; quoted in David R. Hopkins, *Prince and Peasants: Smallpox in History* (Chicago: University of Chicago Press, 1983), p. 281.

Placing blame for disease is important because of its social implications. The drawing of boundaries not only defines the healthy and the sick; it is also an implicit call for the elimination of pollution, the destruction of the sources of disease. Thus blame for disease has justified persecution and destruction. When Jews were labeled as the cause of the Black Death in the fourteenth century, it was not merely an exercise in creating "insider" and "outsider" groups, it was a call for destruction; there followed the murder of entire Jewish communities in York and in Mainz. A similar pattern was evident in the great outbreak of "witch hunting" during the sixteenth and seventeenth centuries. Of the tens of thousands of "witches" burned over two centuries, many were women accused of having caused illness through their black magic.

Blame for disease has also affected medical treatments. When smallpox was associated with immoral behavior, the treatments were often repugnant (for example, a drink made from sheep's dung), on the idea that medicine would drive out evil influence only if its repugnance was in proportion to the sin.[36] But social definitions of disease can also lead to progressive reforms. In the mid-nineteenth century health officers were able to turn their pietistic and class-directed explanations of disease to effective public-health reforms. John Griscom, for example, turned his moral judgments about the degradation of the poor into a plan for the "sanitary regeneration of society."[37]

The way we locate blame for AIDS has implications for its control—through quarantine, education, the allocation of funds for research or health care, compulsory testing or public-health reforms. Moral definitions of responsibility have encouraged discriminatory and coercive policies, even in the face of contrary scientific evidence. Most medical authorities and health-care professionals oppose mandatory AIDS testing,

[36] Hopkins, *Prince and Peasants*, p. 32.
[37] Rosenberg, *No Other Gods*.

but many political leaders, confusing medical goals with their ideological assumptions, continue to insist that specific categories of people—in particular, immigrants, refugees, aliens, and even foreign tourists—should be tested.

Despite the sophisticated scientific understanding underlying concepts of disease in the late twentieth century, we still seek explanations based on behavior, ethnicity, or social stereotypes. We still use disease to protect our social boundaries or to maintain our political ideals. And, at a time when control over disease is limited, we still blame others as a way to protect ourselves. By drawing firm boundaries—that is, by placing blame on "other groups" or on "deviant behavior"— we try to avoid the randomness of disease and dying, to escape from our inherent sense of vulnerability, to exorcise the mortality inherent in the human condition.

II. Science and Health—Possibilities, Probabilities, and Limitations

BY LEWIS THOMAS

U P until just a few years ago, a tour of the exhibition of art works now on display at the Museum of Natural History would have left the impression, in most minds, of events very remote in time, pieces of very ancient history, a strange and disturbing world now well behind us. For the modern mind, especially the everyday modern mind now so adept at dismissing the memories of the great wars of this century with all those deaths, the notion that great numbers of human beings can die all at once from a single cause is as far away and alien as the pyramids. Even more strange is the notion that human death could ever be so visible, so out in the open. Our idea about death is that it takes place privately, in the dark, away from other people. There is something faintly indecent, wrong, about dying in full view of the public.

This is understandable, at least for those of us who live in the Western, industrialized world and have grown to adulthood in the last half of this century. Dying is now the exceptional thing to do, almost an aberration, in our culture. We concede the possibility, even in our bad moments the inevitability, but never before its time. Moreover, that time, the appropriate and acceptable moment, is being pushed further and further into the distance ahead. When the century began, the average life expectancy for Americans and Europeans was around forty-six years; now the life span for a great many of us to bet on will be nearly double that number. Excluding war, of course, in which case all bets are off.

Indeed, the nearest equivalent to the plagues that afflicted human populations in earlier centuries has become, for our own kind of society, dying itself. We know in our bones that we will all die, sooner or later, but we find it harder and harder to put up with the idea; we want the later to be later still. We think of dying as though it were failure, humiliation, losing a game in which there ought to be winners. Many of us take the view that it can indeed be put off, stalled off anyway, by changing the way we live. "Lifestyle" moved into the language by way of its connection with getting sick and dying. We jog, skip, attend aerobic classes, eat certain "food groups" as though food itself was a new kind of medicine, even try to change our thoughts to make our cells sit up and behave like healthy cells; meditation is taken as medication by some of the most ardent meditators. We do these things not so much to keep fit, which is a healthy exercise and good for the mind, but to fend off dying, which is an effort not so good for the mind, maybe in the long run bad for the mind.

A certain worry about death is, of course, nothing new; it is the oldest of normal emotions. But it does seem to me strange that the anxiety has acquired more urgency, and plagued us more in the last years of this peculiar century than ever before, during the very years when most of us have had a good shot at living longer lives than any previous human population.

Partly, I suppose, we fear death more acutely because of this very fact. It never occurred to us, until quite recently, that we had any say at all in the matter; death just came. But now, when it seems that we can put it off, for at least as long as we have in recent decades, why not still longer? If instead of surviving for an average lifetime of three or four decades, as used to be the rule, we can stretch it out to eight or nine, why not fix things so that we keep running for twelve or fifteen, and even then why stop?

But now, at the moment of such high expectations, we are being brought up short, with a glimpse—a brief and early one, to be sure—of what living was like long centuries ago. Just within the past half-dozen years we have been confronted again by the prospect of mortality on a very big scale. And not the dying that used to nag at our minds, the slipping of our finger-hold on life because of the weakness of old age. This time it is the death of our young adults, including in one group some of the most talented and productive, in another group a great many young people born and raised in the deprivation of our most benighted neighborhoods. Moreover, it is already a near certainty that what we are seeing now is only the beginning of something far more menacing: the transition of an epidemic now localized within a minority of the population into a pandemic affecting everyone. We have only to look at the course of events in parts of Africa, where whole settlements are now infected by AIDS. The virus is on the loose in Africa, and there is no reason to hope that it will not spread into the community at large in every other part of the world.

We do not know enough about this extraordinary virus—or, as it is already beginning to appear, this set of extraordinary viruses, all closely related but differing in subtle ways—and we have a great deal to learn. And it seems to me self-evident that the only sure way out of the dilemma must be by research. This is not to say that education and behavioral change will not be valuable in the short run as ways to limit the spread for the time being, to slow down the pandemic for a while. Obviously, we should be instructing all young people in what the virus is and what we already know about how its contagion works, and surely we should be trying whatever we can, including more methadone clinics and the free distribution of sterile needles within the heroin-addicted community. But these are not the answers for the long run. If we are to avert what otherwise lies somewhere ahead, we will have to find out how to kill this virus without killing the cells in which it is lodged, or how to immunize the entire population against the virus, or both. These are scientific problems, very difficult and complex, perhaps the hardest ones ever to confront biomedical science. But at the same time they are nothing like blank mysteries. There has already occurred an exceedingly rapid and encouraging progress in the relatively few laboratories now working on the problem, and it is as close to a certainty as anything I can think of in medicine that the AIDS problem can be solved. The point I hope to make is that the work is only at its beginning, in its early stages, and there is a great deal still to be learned.

A Glance Back

It comes as something of a surprise, even a shock, to realize that we are faced by a brand-new infectious disease about which we understand so little and can therefore *do* so little. Modern medicine has left on the public mind the conviction that we know almost everything about everything. This is as good a time as any to amend that impression. There are, here and there, pieces of evidence that biomedical science—as we like to call the enterprise, thus combining the now-hardening science of biology with the prestige of medicine—good as it is, is perhaps not entitled to all the credit it gets from the general public.

It needs a glance back to see what happened to improve our longevity. And then, perhaps, a quick and speculative look ahead.

Science had a hand in our betterment, to be sure, and medicine played a modest hand of its own, but nothing like the decisive role that is assumed in some quarters. To read the papers, you might think that medicine turned itself into a full-fledged science all on its own just in the past century, and that is why we now live longer than we did in the eighteenth or nineteenth century. This is an agreeable thought for the minds of doctors, but hard to document. It is true that the basic biomedical science in microbiology and immunology, starting a little over 100 years ago, eventually brought along the applied sciences of immunization and antibiotic therapy. In its new capacity to prevent or cure the major infectious diseases of human beings in Western societies, medicine could now lay a fair claim to being scientific, but only in part. And even here, in what everyone would acknowledge to be the greatest therapeutic triumph of modern medicine, questions about the actual role of science can be raised. Typhoid fever and cholera had already become rare, even exotic diseases in most parts of the industrialized world long before the emergence of antibiotics, thanks mostly to better sanitation, good plumbing, improved nutrition and less crowded living quarters—in short, a higher standard of living. The morbidity and mortality from tuberculosis was well on its way down, long before the discovery of streptomycin, INH, rifampin and the rest had opened the way to rational treatment, and the accomplishment was the result of a combination of old-fashioned public-health measures plus a spontaneous decrease in susceptibility to TB infection among a better-fed, sturdier population. Rheumatic fever and valvular heart disease had already begun to decline before the introduction of penicillin prophylaxis.

One of the most spectacular triumphs was, of course, the virtual elimination of tertiary syphilis. I have lately been asking around among my neurological colleagues in the New York and Boston academic medical centers, and have found no one who has seen a patient with general paresis in the last ten years. This malignant disorder of the mind, which filled more state hospital beds than schizophrenia when I was a medical student, has very nearly vanished. But how did this happen? Was it the result of meticulous case-finding and early penicillin treatment of all cases of primary and secondary syphilis (of which there is still an abundance in all our cities)? I rather doubt it, especially considering the debilitated condition of most of today's municipal and county health departments. Then how to explain it? With early syphilis still a common, everyday disease, much of it subsiding into latent syphilis without treatment as always happened in the past, why are we not seeing tertiary syphilis, especially syphilis of the brain?

My theory is that it happened because of science, but a misapplication of science. Since it first came on the medical marketplace, penicillin has been scandalously overprescribed and overused. Most patients with upper-respiratory-tract infections or unaccounted-for febrile illnesses receive penicillin at one time or another, probably in doses sufficient to eliminate spirochetes wherever they are. In the virtual aerosol of penicillin that has affected whole nations in the past forty years, tertiary syphilis has, quite by accident, been almost eliminated.

Something like this perhaps also accounts for the increasing rarity of rheumatic heart disease in recent decades. The group A beta-hemolytic streptococcus is still among us, but its capacity to launch the old epidemics of throat infections among our schoolchildren may now be sharply restricted by the ever-presence of penicillin being used for the wrong reasons. If so, it is hard to call this science, but never mind, it works anyway.

The incidence of fatal coronary thrombosis in the United States has changed dramatically, and for the better, since the 1950s, dropping year by year to an aggregate decrease of around 20 percent. No one seems to know why this happened, which is not in itself surprising since no one really knows for sure what the underlying mechanism responsible for coronary disease is. In the circumstance, everyone is free to provide one's own theory, depending on one's opinion about the mechanism. You can claim, if you like, that there has been enough reduction in the dietary intake of saturated fat, nationwide, to make the difference, although I think you'd have a hard time proving it. Or, if you prefer, you can attribute it to the epidemic of jogging, but I think that the fall in incidence of coronary disease had already begun before jogging became a national mania. Or, if you are among those who believe that an excessively competitive personality strongly influences the incidence of this disease, you might assert that more of us have become calmer and less combative since the 1950s, and I suppose you could back up the claim by simply listing the huge numbers of new mental-health professionals, counselors, lifestyle authorities, and various health gurus who have appeared in our midst in recent years. But I doubt it, just as I doubt their effectiveness in calming us all down.

My own theory is that the 20 percent drop in American coronary disease was the result of commercial television, which appeared in the early 1950s and has made a substantial part of its living ever since through the incessant advertising, all day and all night, of household remedies for headache and back pain, all containing aspirin. One plausible result of this may have been the maintenance, down the years, of a national level of blood salicylate set at an optimal range for the inhibition of prostaglandin synthetase and, as a result, a 20 percent reduction in platelet stickiness. If I am right, we might predict an upturn in the incidence now that aspirin is having a rather bad press and variants of Tylenol are in fashion.

My contention is that we do indeed have some science in the practice of medicine, but not anything like enough, and we have a great distance to go. Indeed, most of what is regarded as high science in medicine is actually a set of technologies for diagnostic precision—the CAT scan, NMR, and many exquisite refinements of our methods for detecting biochemical abnormalities of one sort or another. But these have not yet been matched by any comparable transformations in therapy. We are still confronted by the chronic disablements of an aging population, lacking any clear understanding of the mechanisms of these diseases—dementia, for instance, or diabetes or cirrhosis or arthritis or stroke and all the rest on a long list—and without knowing the underlying mechanisms we lack new therapeutic approaches. To be sure, we do have some spectacular surgical achievements in the headlines, the transplantation of hearts, kidneys, livers, and the like, but these are what I have called halfway technologies, brought in to shore things up after the still-unexplained diseases of these organs have run their course. And these measures, plus the new advances in diagnostic precision, account for a large part of the escalating costs of health care today. It seems obvious, to me anyway, that the only practical policy for bringing down those costs will be by more and more basic research in biomedical science, in the hope and expectation that we can then begin to understand, at a deep level, the underlying events in human disease. Sooner or later I am confident that this will be accomplished, and I hope for the sooner. This is the mission, by the way, of the National Institutes of Health, and I hope nobody tries to disturb, for any political purpose, the functioning of this extraordinary institution, either by "privatizing" it, as some ideologues have openly proposed, or by micromanaging its affairs, as congressional committees are sometimes tempted to do. I have thought many times in recent years that if you are looking around for some piece of solid evidence that government really can work brilliantly well—and these days many are indeed looking despairingly for such evidences—take a glance at NIH, in its singular way the finest social invention of the twentieth century.

One reason why medical history is not much taught in medical schools is that so much of it is an embarrassment. During all the millennia of its existence as a profession, all the way back to its origins in shamanism, the public expectations of medicine have been high, demanding, and difficult to meet. First among the demands was to recognize the existence of a disease, explain it, and then make it go away. For most of its history, medicine has been unable to do any of these things, and its sole advantage to a patient seeking help lay in the doctor's capacity to provide reassurance and then to stand by while the illness, whatever, ran its course. The doctor's real role during all those centuries was more like that of a professional friend, someone at the bedside, standing by. When he was called a therapist, it was more in the etymological sense of the original Greek *therapon*: Patroclus was *therapon* to Achilles, part servant, part friend; he stood by him in his troubles, listened to his complaints, advised him when he could, put up with him, finally even died for him. Therapy was a much more powerful word for the ancient Greeks than it is today, and somewhere along the line it was picked up by the doctors. In its ancient meaning, it carries inside all the obligations that medicine and the other health professions have for patients with AIDS: to stand by, to do whatever can be done, to comfort, and to run all the risks that doctors have always run in times of plague.

When I arrived at Harvard Medical School in 1933, nobody talked about therapeutics as though it were a coherent medical discipline, in the sense that pharmacology is today. To be sure, there were a few things to learn about: digitalis for heart failure, insulin, liver extract for pernicious anemia, vitamin B for pellagra, a few others. By and large, we were instructed not to meddle. Our task was to learn all that was known about the natural history of disease so that we could make an accurate diagnosis, and a reasonably probabilistic prognosis. That done, our function as doctors would be to enlist the best possible nursing care, explain matters to the patient and family, and stand by.

Moreover, we were taught that this was not only the very best kind of medicine—not to meddle—it was the way medicine would be for the rest of our lives. None of us, certainly not any of the medical students, had the faintest notion that our profession would ever be any different from what it was in the 1930s. We were totally unprepared for the upheaval that came with the sulfonamides, and then with penicillin. We could hardly believe our eyes on seeing that bacteria could be killed off without at the same time killing the patient. It was not just an amazement, it was a revolution.

That made two revolutions. The first, that the medical treatments in common use for all the centuries before our time didn't really work, did more harm than good, and had to be given up, left us with almost nothing to do to alter the course or outcome of a human illness. And then the second, that a form of treatment based on fundamental research, tested in experimental animals, then tested in controlled experiments in human beings, was possible. Medicine, it seemed, was off and running. Nothing seemed beyond reach. If we could cure streptococcal septicemia, epidemic meningitis, subacute bacterial endocarditis, tuberculosis, tertiary syphilis, typhoid fever, even typhus fever, was there anything we could not do? Easy one hand, we thought.

By the 1950s it was beginning to become clear that solving all the rest of medicine's problems was going to be a lot harder than we had thought. Some of us had overlooked the fact that the conquest of bacterial infection and the success in immunizing against certain viral diseases had not simply fallen into the lap of medicine. These things could not have happened at all without the most penetrating insight into the underlying mechanisms of the diseases we were able to treat or prevent so effectively. Not to say that we had much comprehension of how a meningococcus goes about producing meningitis, or how a pneumococcus does its special work in the human lung. These were blank mysteries, and to some extent the mechanisms of pathogenesis remain mysteries today. But what we did know were bits of crucial information: the names and shapes and some of the metabolic habits of the microorganisms involved, the specific pathologic changes they produced in human tissues, and the ways in which they spread through human communities. This information had not dropped into our laps. It came as the outcome of decades of what we would be calling basic biological science if it were going on today. Without the research in microbiology and immunology done in those decades, we could never have entered that first period of modern therapeutic medicine.

Now things are beginning to change. A problem like cancer, which seemed simply unapproachable in the early 1970s, too profound even to make good guesses about, has turned suddenly into the liveliest, most exciting and competitive, and among the most elusive puzzles in all of biology. Instead of appearing to be a hundred different diseases, each requiring eventually its own individual solution, it now seems more likely that a single, centrally placed genetic anomaly will be found as the cause of all human cancers. The new information, coming in as cascades of surprise from laboratories all round the world, will almost surely lead to novel therapeutic and preventive approaches that cannot be predicted at the present time.

There is something of the same excitement and anticipation within the rapidly expanding community of neurobiologists, keeping in the same close touch with each other across all international boundaries. The brain has been transformed within just the past few years from a computer-like instrument of unimaginable complexity to a system governed by chemical messages and run by the specific receptors of scores, more likely hundreds, of short peptide chains of command.

Much of what is now happening in both cancer and brain research is the outcome of basic research that had neither of these problems in mind when the work was started, even when the definitive aspects of the work were well under way. The new field of molecular genetics began to catch glimpses of its potential when the restriction enzymes were discovered, and once the technology of recombinant DNA had evolved to the point where specific molecular probes were at hand, it became clear that the most powerful methods for studying the deep functions of cancer cells were also at hand. Meanwhile, the new technique of cell fusion had led to the development of hybridomas, and monoclonal antibodies had become indispensable for the study of gene products and cell surface antigens. But the people whose work made these techniques possible were not, at the outset of their work, aware that they were putting together a totally new set of approaches to the cancer problem.

Early on, nobody engaged in the work could have predicted how it would turn out or where it would lead, nor can they predict the future benefits today, only that the work is engrossing and fascinating, and filled with surprises yet to come.

This is the way it will go for the rest of medicine, if fundamental biomedical research continues at its present pace and scope. The dementias of the aged, coronary artery disease, arthritis, stroke, schizophrenia and the manic-depressive psychoses, chronic nephritis, cirrhosis, pulmonary fibrosis, multiple sclerosis—any disease you care to name—will be opened up for closer scrutiny by discoveries still unpredictable in biology itself. The information needed for the future cannot be planned by committees or commissions, and there is no way for bureaucracies to decide which pieces of information are needed first, or at what time. In basic science the shots can never be called in advance—or by definition the enterprise is not basic science.

This sounds an optimistic way of looking at the future of medicine, for what I am predicting is that no human disease is any longer so strange a mystery that its underlying mechanism cannot be understood or got at. There are some who will quarrel with this view of things, arguing that I am oversimplifying matters of great complexity. They will say, they do say, that the idea of single causes for disease is outdated and wrong, that people who talk about single causes are influenced too much by the infectious diseases. Today's chronic ailments, they will assert, especially the chronic diseases of aging, do not have single causes, they are multifactorial, whole systems of things gone wrong. The environment itself is what needs fixing, along with lifestyle, diet, exercise, and a new kind of human personality to boot.

Maybe so, but I doubt it. I do not doubt that a good many influences affect the incidence and severity of human disease. Pneumococcal pneumonia is quite a different disease when it occurs in a chronic alcoholic, or when it afflicts a very old person, or a person with immunodeficiency. But the pneumococcus is still at the center of things, the chairman of the board. I think there will be a chairman of the board, perhaps at the head of a whole committee of other mechanisms in the senile dementias, or in schizophrenia, or cirrhosis, or all the rest. And once identified, he can be got at, just as the spirochete of syphilis, running what seems to me the most complicated, multiorgan, multitissue, multimechanism of all the human diseases I have ever learned about, can be got at. Once got at, the simple act of lifting out the spirochete results in the switching off of all the other events. There is no good explanation for this, but it is, I believe, the way things work in human disease.

The AIDS Problem

It is this approach, now getting underway but needing much more expansion, that is needed for the AIDS problem. Through the efforts of NIH, the Pasteur Institute, and a few other laboratories here and abroad, an intelligent investment is already being made—still on a modest scale considering the necessity—in scientific research on the biology of AIDS and the HIV virus. Considering that the virus turned up only a half-dozen or so years ago, and that it is one of the most complex and baffling organisms on earth, the progress that has already been made in the laboratories working on it is an astonishment. I have never observed, in a long lifetime looking at biomedical research, anything to touch it. If this disease had first appeared ten or fifteen years ago, before the research technologies of molecular biology had developed the marvelous tool of recombinant DNA, we would still be completely stuck, unable even to make intelligent guesses about the cause of AIDS. Thanks to the new methods, which emerged from entirely basic research having nothing at all to do with any medical problem, we now know more about the structure, molecular composition, behavior and target cells than we know about any other virus in the world. The work, in short, is going beautifully. But it is still in its early stages, and there is an unknown distance still to go. At the moment, there seem to be three lines of research holding the most promise, and there is a conspicuous shortfall already in the funds needed for each of these lines.

One approach, the most direct of the three but also the most difficult and unpredictable, is in the field of pharmacology. We need a new class of antiviral drugs, capable of killing off the virus inside all the invaded cells without killing the cells themselves. These drugs must be comparable in their effectiveness to the antibiotics which came into medicine for use against bacterial infections fifty years ago. We already have a few partially active drugs; these may turn out to be the primitive precursors of such a class, AZT for example, but their effectiveness is still incomplete, temporarily palliative at best, and their toxicity is unacceptable. However, there are no theoretical reasons against the development of decisively effective antivirals, including drugs to stop the replication of retroviruses like HIV. What is urgently needed, indispensable in fact, is some new and very deep information about the intimate details of retroviruses and the enzyme systems that enable them to penetrate and multiply within the target cells that are their specialty in life. In short, more basic research of the most fundamental kind.

Second, we need an abundance of new information about the human immune system. The only imaginable way to prevent the continuing spread of HIV—even when and if we have in hand an antiviral drug that really works to control infection in individual cases—will be by producing a vaccine. What this means is that more information is needed concerning the molecular labels at the surface of this virus, and which among these labels represents a point of vulnerability for an immune response. Since it is already known that this particular virus has the strange property of changing its own labels from time to time, even the labeling of the same HIV virus isolated at different stages of the disease in the same patient, it will be no easy task to produce a vaccine. A small number of vaccine trials are already underway in small cohorts of human subjects. There is no reason to be optimistic about these at the present time, nor is there any feasible way to hurry things up. With luck, a lot of luck, some laboratory may succeed in identifying for sure a stable and genuinely vulnerable target molecule in HIV, and then a vaccine will be feasible. But as things stand now, there can be no assurance that a vaccine prepared against this year's crop of HIV viruses will be any more effective against the viruses at large five years hence than that an influenza vaccine prepared several years ago will be of any use against next winter's outbreak of flu.

A third line of research involves the human immune system itself, the primary victim of the AIDS virus. Actually, most if not all patients with AIDS die from other kinds of infection, not because of any direct, lethal action of the virus itself. The process is a subtle one, more like endgame in chess. What the virus does, selectively and with exquisite precision, is to take out the population of lymphocytes that carry responsibilities for defending the body against all sorts of microbes in the world outside, most of which are harmless to normal humans. In a sense, the patients are not dying because of the HIV virus, they are being killed by great numbers of other bacteria and viruses that can now swarm into a defenseless host. Research is needed to gain a deeper understanding of the biology of the immune cells, in the hope of preserving them or replacing them by transplantation of normal immune cells. This may be necessary even if we are successful in finding drugs to destroy the virus itself; by the time this has been accomplished in some patients, it may be that the immune system has already been wiped out, and the only open course will be to replace these cells.

This had already become one of the liveliest fields in basic immunology long before the appearance of AIDS, and what is now needed is an intensification of the research. In my own view (perhaps biased because of my own background in immunology) it is the most urgent and promising of all current approaches to the AIDS problem.

To sum up, AIDS is first and last a scientific research matter, only to be solved by basic investigation in good laboratories. The research that has been done in the last few years has been elegant and highly productive, with results that tell us one sure thing: it is a soluble problem even though an especially complex and difficult one. No one can predict, at this stage, how it will turn out or where the really decisive answers to our questions will be found, but the possibilities are abundant and the prospects are bright. It is particularly encouraging that the basic research most needed is being conducted by collaborative groups in both academic and industrial establishments. This is a new phenomenon in this country, well worth noting in the present context. Up until just recently, the past decade or so, the university laboratories and their counterparts in the pharmaceutical industry tended to hold apart from each other, indeed rather looked down their noses at each other. It took the biological revolution of the 1970s, and specifically the new technologies of recombinant DNA and monoclonal antibodies, to bring the scientists from both communities into a close intellectual relationship, with each side now recognizing that the other could offer invaluable contributions to the research on ways to intervene in the mechanisms of human disease. And now, as the science moves along from one surprise to the next, especially in the fields of molecular biology and virology, the lines that we used to think of as separating basic and applied research into two distinct categories have become more and more blurred. Academic and industry scientists recognize that they are really in the same line of work, and research partnerships of a new kind are being set up all over the place, and the scientists, by and large, are moving as fast as they can. It is already clear that there is not enough talent to go round. However, I take this to be an exceedingly healthy transformation in our institutions. The response must be the recruiting and training of more bright young people for the work ahead.

I should say a few words here about the possibilities for spin-offs from AIDS research. Briefly, they are endless. The immunologic defect produced by the HIV virus brings about an increased vulnerability to Kaposi's sarcoma, and the same class of immune cells may play an important role in the defense of humans against many other, perhaps all, types of cancer. The dementias that occur in terminal AIDS infection resemble other types of human dementia, and new information about the former should shed light on the latter. If we can learn how to block the HIV retroviruses without killing the cells in which they are lodged, we will find ourselves armed with a new, more general class of antiviral drugs, of very general usefulness. It used to be said as a truism in medical school, long ago when I was a medical student, that if we could ever reach a full understanding of the events that occurred in the human body as the result of one single disease, syphilis, we would know everything in the world about medicine. This is the hunch I have today about AIDS.

It is obvious that the science that is needed for the AIDS problem in the years just ahead will be possible only with the support of large expenditures of public money. The commitment will demand public support, obviously. But I do wish, and fervently hope, that it can somehow be taken out of politics itself. AIDS is not, emphatically not, a political problem. Questions about testing people for the virus, and whom to test, even how to test, and how to preserve confidentiality, are proper questions for the public-health professionals who have known for years how to do this kind of thing, and they are not proper questions for politicians running for office. AIDS is a complicated scientific puzzle, as complex as any yet faced by biomedical science, and more urgent than any other I can think of. It is, in short, an emergency for science, the best science to be done by the best scientists we can assemble, in as international an effort as we can bring into being, and as quickly as possible.

III. Case Histories— An Introduction

BY BARBARA
GUTMANN
ROSENKRANTZ

PLAGUES, as everyone knows, lead to the erection of barriers—*cordons sanitaires* and quarantines that separate the sick from the well with the intention of enhancing both the letter and spirit of security. Less often considered is the measure of confidence lent to new voices of authority in time of plague. Public concern about the dangers of AIDS and the social impact of this unanticipated epidemic have, for example, prompted the media to ask historians about plagues of the past. Most often the question asked is quite general: "Are there precedents for the AIDS epidemic?" And most often historians shape their answers to meet the limitations of their own professional knowledge. We learn that outbreaks of bubonic plague in Europe and England from the late fifteenth to the late seventeenth centuries occurred in the context of constrained economic as well as scientific resources, and that religious belief shaped the responses of those in authority as well as popular sentiment. And historians of the nineteenth century explain that when cholera swept from the East to the West, an environment in which population density generated public sensitivity to social disorders paved the way for new concepts of disease causation and transmission. But not surprisingly, the question of whether there were "precursors" to AIDS remains unanswered, and the notion that natural history or human social history generates precedents revealing predictable patterns seems at best inadequate. One fundamental and striking novelty of the late twentieth century is the expectation of near-perfect protection from contagious disease.

The papers that follow approach the history of past diseases from different perspectives, but the authors—two historians and a scientist—share the view that there is much to be learned about the order of human societies and values from popular and medical responses to epidemic diseases of the distant—and not so distant—past. Paul Slack, Baruch S. Blumberg, and Allan M. Brandt also indicate that the impact of epidemic disease has been affected by human actions, sometimes by interventions that are deliberate as in the effect of quarantine, but also in instances where the course of epidemic disease is altered as a consequence of less direct intention, as in reaction to altered nutritional status.

These interactions of man and microorganism are not, of course, interactions that have patiently awaited recent developments in the biomedical human sciences, nor have observations and explanations of the complex interplay of man and disease waited for contemporary historical research. The papers in this section associate the varied history of human responses to the threats of dangerous disease with more general social and moral values. Despite the distance of the bubonic plague or cholera in time and feelings, the historian's skill in restructuring what Slack calls "the interpretive system" that provided peoples of the past with the emotional and intellectual apparatus for giving meaning to experience shows how understanding and confidence were constructed in the absence of scientific knowledge. Is there in the historian's reconstruction of dread disease an implied analogy to the current threat of AIDS in the context of its fatal course, resistant to known therapies? The answer is, most firmly, no. The personal and public uncertainties and accommodations that surrounded much contagious disease even half a century ago seem intolerable today in the context of preventive and therapeutic achievements. If the AIDS epidemic has made us conscious of the limitations of current social and scientific controls of contagion, it is perhaps inevitable, but certainly misleading, to draw simple lessons about ecologic and moral imbalance from the unanticipated eruption of a new and lethal disease.

Through these carefully researched accounts we are exposed not only to a modest understanding of the interaction of man and microbe in history but also to the contemporary historian's caution not to distort the impact of the explanatory system that fit into the world of Daniel Defoe with the implication that seventeenth-century Englishmen made sense of fearsome events much as we do today. The ordinary vices that tempt us to make simple sense of history are, not surprisingly, embedded in our culture. They offer the same temptations that we face in mounting resistance to the uncertainties of epidemic disease: the vice of "whiggery," through which we celebrate linear progress and reassuringly demonstrate how evil is overwhelmed by good, and the vice of relativism, which separates the event from its context so we may conclude that nothing has really changed.

But our anxieties about technological fixes and our expectations of scientific medicine contrast starkly with past reliance on diffuse sources of power to relieve the disorder and distress of disease. One can imagine that the historian's authority at one time eased mortal terrors when experience was infused with "meanings," which are now more apparent as "symbolic" because they have lost their immediate explanatory power. But scientific knowledge does not suck social meanings out of disease leaving an objectified hull, and the historian is not a surrogate for the scientific expert in our time. These papers on bubonic plague, venereal diseases, and hepatitis B prompt us to search for the elements that continue to shape the social and personal meanings of disease, and in particular to consider the history of circumstances in which the relationship between scientific knowledge and authority has acquired power over uncertainties in our time of plague.

Hepatitis B Virus and the Carrier Problem*

BARUCH S. BLUMBERG

This conference is dedicated to the notion that we are children of history and can learn about the future by studying the past. This process also teaches us that we usually don't do so; but that shouldn't deter us from examining the history of disease in order to find directions for contemporary health problems—for example, the current tragic epidemic of AIDS.

My plan today is to discuss the experience with a worldwide pandemic of infection with the hepatitis B virus (HBV), starting from about the time that the virus was identified.[1] Many of the same ethical, social, psychological, and research problems that have arisen with other infectious disease epidemics have been encountered with HBV, but each has a character of its own. I'll attempt to point out some of these problems as they apply to AIDS and other diseases as the narrative unfolds.

HBV and HIV

HBV has many similarities to the virus that is considered to be the cause of AIDS, the human immunodeficiency virus (HIV). HIV is a RNA retrovirus, one that replicates using a step in which the RNA of the virus makes DNA using the enzyme reverse transcriptase to do so. HBV is classified as a

[1] B. S. Blumberg, "Australia Antigen and the Biology of Hepatitis B," *Science* 197 (1977): 17–25.

DNA virus. However, in its replication process, HBV also utilizes a reverse transcriptase to make DNA from RNA. In addition, HBV has epidemiologic characteristics in common with HIV. Many of the groups that are at high risk for infection with HIV are also at risk for HBV: male homosexuals, transfused patients and patients who receive certain blood products (e.g., hemophilia patients), drug abusers, the newborn children of infected mothers, and certain populations in Africa. There are, however, exceptions. For example, HBV infection is very common in China, Japan, India, and other countries in Asia, but HIV is rare.

HBV has an affinity for the liver; it can seriously impair liver function and lead to yellow jaundice, the most striking finding in the disease. Many cases result in an acute disease which can be disabling but usually progresses to a complete recovery. Some acute cases, however, develop chronic infection and chronic liver disease which can cause disability and shorten life expectancy. In addition, many people are occultly infected with HBV and become chronic carriers of the virus. There are estimated to be about 200 million carriers of HBV in the world, most of them in Africa and Asia. There are about 1 million carriers in the United States. Carriers remain asymptomatic for many years, but some will eventually suffer from chronic liver disease and, particularly in Asia and Africa, are at relatively high risk for the development of primary cancer of the liver. In these regions, cancer of the liver is one of the most common cancers and a problem of public-health proportions.

There are important differences between HIV and HBV. HBV has been around for a long time; it may have been noted in the Egyptian and Indian Ayurvedic texts and in the Babylonian Talmud. Many indigenous medical systems contain remedies for the treatment of jaundice, some of which was probably due to HBV infection. HIV, on the other hand, appears to have been introduced recently—perhaps in the 1970s—and was rare until the present decade.

The diseases are perceived differently by the public; because of its high fatality rate, AIDS is far more feared. However, worldwide, more people are made ill or die as a consequence of HBV infection. Another important difference is that there is a very effective and safe vaccine to prevent infection with HBV; at present, none is available for HIV.

Discovery of Hepatitis B Virus

In the mid 1960s, we discovered that HBV could be detected in blood by the use of a reactant present in the blood of patients who had received large numbers of transfusions. Apparently, some transfusion units had contained HBV, and the patients had developed an antibody against it which could be used to detect the virus in other people's blood. By a strange irony, the blood of people who had already been exposed to the virus and developed an antibody against it could be used to detect the virus present in donors' blood and prevent its use to infect others.

In a relatively short time, sensitive methods were developed to screen donor blood and detect asymptomatic carriers of HBV. Prior to this discovery, hepatitis following transfusions with blood from carriers of HBV was very common, particularly with the introduction in the 1950s of surgical procedures such as open-heart surgery and kidney transplantation that required large amounts of blood. In some hospitals where these heroic surgical procedures were performed, as many as 50 percent of the patients became infected, and many of them became seriously ill. Therefore, as soon as it was realized that hepatitis screening would considerably decrease the frequency of posttransfusion hepatitis, many blood banks established testing as a routine procedure, and it soon became a requirement for all hospitals and blood banks. The incidence of posttransfusion hepatitis due to HBV has decreased dramatically.[2]

[2] B. S. Blumberg, "The Discovery of Hepatitis B Virus," in *Legionellosis*, vol. 2, ed. S. M. Katz (Boca Raton, Fla.: CRC Press, Inc., 1985), pp. 171–176.

There was an interesting and curious consequence of the
development of tests for the detection of carriers. It was
quickly realized that they were of great commercial importance, since all donor bloods required testing. The medical-
diagnostics industry developed rapid, sensitive, and reliable
tests for the virus which required large amounts of the human
antibody. We became particularly aware of this when we were
visited by a patient with hemophilia, Mr. Ted Slavin, whose
blood we had tested.[3] He had received hundreds of
transfusions of human blood and had developed high titers of
antibody to the surface antigen of HBV (anti-HBs). During
most of his life, his blood disease had been a terrible burden to
him; he was an energetic and intelligent man, but often when
he achieved success in his business life, he was thwarted by a
recurrence of bleeding. With the development of the test, the
situation was reversed. His blood was now a source of wealth,
since he could sell it at a high price to the reagent
manufacturers. He formed his own company (with the
wonderful name of "Essential Biologicals") and later was able
to obtain a senior position in a larger company. He
imaginatively explored methods for capitalizing on this
resource. He attempted to form a consortium of hemophilia
patients, modeled along the lines of the organization of
oil-producing countries (OPEC), and considered the possibility
of treating his blood as a nonrenewable resource, thereby
entitling him to the depletion allowance tax exemption granted
to oil and gas producers. He very generously donated to us
large quantities of his plasma, which we used extensively in our
research over the course of many years and have preserved as
a form of memorial to this remarkable man.

[3] B. S. Blumberg, I. Millman, W. T. London, and other members of the Division of
Clinical Research, Fox Chase Cancer Center, Philadelphia, Pa., "Ted Slavin's Blood
and the Development of HBV Vaccine: Letter to the Editor," *New England Journal of
Medicine* 312 (1985): 189.

Blood Screening

Medicine is filled with strange and unexpected outcomes. It often seems that as soon as a problem is solved, it raises others, and every answer raises even more questions.

As the testing programs were mounted, we began to hear disquieting stories about people who had been identified as carriers during the course of the blood-bank screening and other testing programs.[4] About 12 million units of blood are transfused in the United States yearly, and all donors, plus others, would, in due course, be tested. For example, we were consulted by a nurse whose blood had been tested and found to carry HBV. She was told by her employers that she could no longer work at the hospital. Another incident occurred during a visit to a country which at that time had a military government. I had been asked by the medical authorities if applicants for admission to medical school should be screened and those found to be carriers refused admission; the same question was asked in regard to admission to officer training schools. (I recommended against it.) There even had been a suggestion in the medical press that nursing students should be examined before graduation and those found to be carriers refused permission to practice.[5]

A particularly difficult issue arose in respect to adoption of children from Vietnam. Many orphans had been brought to the United States and placed for adoption. What if these children had been screened and some of them found to be carriers? Would this affect their chance of adoption? Would a single blood test determine the fate of a young child? The Public Health Service decided not to test these orphans for HBV as a condition of entry.

What we appeared to be witnessing was the development of

---

[4] B. S. Blumberg, "Bioethical Questions Related to Hepatitis B Antigen," *American Journal of Clinical Pathology* 65 (1976): 848–853.

[5] C. A. C. Ross, "Recommends that Nurses Who Are Carriers Not Be Certified," *British Medical Journal* 1 (1975): 95.

a stigmatized class of individuals identified by a single blood test. There was clearly a conflict between individual rights and public-health issues, and this was happening at a time when we had incomplete knowledge about the transmission and possible protective measures against HBV. Clearly, more research was required; but what was to be done in the meanwhile? On the one hand, we knew that transmission by means of transfusion of the blood of carriers was quite common. In this case, the issue was clear. There was an obvious advantage to the patient and to society in preventing the use of the carrier blood, and the disadvantages to the donor were slight; he or she was simply told not to donate blood in the future. But the advantages and disadvantages in respect to methods of transmission other than by transfusion were not so clear. It was obvious that person-to-person transmission could occur, but this was mainly conjugal and within the household, and it did not appear to be a great risk to people with only a casual interaction with the carrier. There were about 1 million carriers in the United States, and if the virus were very infectious one would have expected to see many more cases of transmission than were known to occur. It appeared that some carriers were prone to transmit HBV while others were not, and at this stage of our knowledge there was no method for distinguishing between them. There were observations on health-care personnel who were known to be carriers; there appeared to be a very low risk that they would transmit the virus to their patients.[6] (Dentists, however, appeared to be an exception.[7]) In any case, even if carriers were detected in the general population, it wasn't at all clear what one would tell them to do. There is no advantage to a screening program if there is no obvious consequent action of a constructive nature.

[6] H. J. Alter and others, "Health-care Workers Positive for Hepatitis B Surface Antigen, Are Their Contacts at Risk?," *New England Journal of Medicine* 292 (1975): 454–457.

[7] J. W. Mosley and others, "Hepatitis B Virus Infection in Dentists," *New England Journal of Medicine* 293 (1975): 729–734.

To summarize, in the case of person-to-person transmission, the advantages and disadvantages of screening were difficult to evaluate. There was no practical medical or public-health advantage to detecting the carriers since little could be done after detection (with some exceptions) and there was a very clear disadvantage to the carrier, who might lose employment, face social ostracism, and undergo other disadvantages with no compensatory advantages. There were, as already discussed, clear advantages to blood-donor screening. An ethical judgment was required; it was decided that donor blood would be screened but general screening programs would not be instituted until research was completed that would allow more intelligent handling of the results.

That appears to be what happened. Screening of donor blood was widely accepted (it is required by law or regulation in many jurisdictions in the United States and other countries) but general screening was not widely used. There was, however, an acceleration in research. The results of this completely changed the situation so that in some circumstances the ethical situation was not completely reversed and it became beneficial to screen the general population. What was the research that led to these changes?

Vaccine

An important development was the introduction of a vaccine which protects against HBV. My colleague at the Fox Chase Cancer Center, Dr. Irving Millman, and I developed a method for producing the vaccine from blood.[8] This was possible because HBV is an unusual human virus in that carriers have in their blood large numbers of particles which contain only the

[8] I. Millman, "The Development of the Hepatitis B Vaccine," in I. Millman, T. K. Eisenstein, and B. S. Blumberg, eds., *Hepatitis B: The Virus, the Disease and the Vaccine* (New York: Plenum, 1984), pp. 137–147.

outside coat of the virus (hepatitis B surface antigen, HBsAg). HBsAg particles are not infectious and cannot cause disease, but they can be used as a vaccine. To produce the vaccine, they are separated from the relatively few whole virus particles in the blood and treated to kill any virus which might remain. With the addition of preservatives and adjuvant, this material itself constituted the vaccine. It appears that the virus manufactures within the cells of one host a "vaccine" which could be used to protect other people who had never been infected.

There were amusing conjectures that arose from this unique method of producing a vaccine. Carriers of HBV were the source of the vaccine. One could envision the situation sometime in the future when the virus would disappear. Hence the source of the vaccine would be gone just about the time it was no longer needed! These conjectures are redundant, however, since the vaccine can now be made by recombinant DNA methods (the first human vaccine to be commercially manufactured in this manner) and the carriers are no longer the sole source of starting material.

Arrangements were made for the development and manufacture of the vaccine; it was eventually tested in several large field trials in New York, San Francisco and elsewhere.[9] It was found to be very effective; more than 90 percent of those vaccinated are protected. It is also very safe. The blood-derived vaccine has now been used by several million people and there have been no reports of detrimental side effects. It is being used widely in the United States but even more so in Asia, Africa, and southern Europe, where HBV is a much more serious problem. There are now national programs in the People's Republic of China and several other countries for vaccination of all newborn children.

An interesting feature of the research and application pro-

---

[9] W. Szmuness, C. E. Stevens, and E. J. Harley, "Hepatitis B Vaccine: Demonstration of Efficacy in a Controlled Clinical Trial in a High-Risk Population in the United States," *New England Journal of Medicine* 303 (1980): 833–841.

grams for HBV was the modest media attention it attracted. Very few of the developments were carried as front-page items, and even when the blood screening and vaccine programs were introduced, there was only moderate media interest. Several of the ethical problems received inside-page coverage, but little more. In contrast, practically every facet of the AIDS problem is newsworthy. This, again, probably arises from the different perceptions the public has of the diseases; AIDS is greatly feared, and hepatitis much less so.

There was an ironic consequence of this "fear gap." As noted, the HBV vaccine is prepared from blood, and a fear arose that it might transmit HIV, which is known to be carried in the blood. In a series of studies, it was conclusively demonstrated that this did not happen.[10] The method of producing the vaccine includes several steps that would kill all known viruses and, in particular, HIV, which is not a very hardy organism. There was still resistance to the use of the vaccine. Dentists were particularly prone to infection with HBV since they ordinarily did not use gloves as surgeons do.[11] Despite the significant exposure they had, there was not a wide acceptance of the vaccine or the use of gloves by the dental profession. When the AIDS epidemic began, dentists were particularly concerned. It has subsequently been shown that they are at extremely low risk of developing AIDS. Despite this low risk, dentists are now using gloves and masks, which has the secondary and more important effect of protecting them from HBV. Providence works in strange ways.

Changes in the Ethics of Screening

With the introduction of the vaccine, the ethical problems

[10] B. Poisz and others, "Hepatitis B Vaccine: Evidence Confirming Lack of AIDS Transmission," *Morbidity and Mortality Weekly Report* 33 (1985): 685–687.

[11] J. W. Mosley and E. White, "Viral Hepatitis as an Occupational Hazard of Dentists," *Journal of the American Dental Association* 90 (1975): 992–997.

changed and it now became advantageous to detect carriers. Most of the person-to-person transmission was within families. We could screen populations with a high frequency of HBV carriers and then recommend vaccination for all family and household members of the identified carriers.

A particularly vulnerable group for infection were the newborn children of carrier mothers. In Japan and elsewhere in Asia, if the mother were a carrier, then the newborn had an extremely high risk of becoming infected and remaining a carrier for an indefinite time. However, vaccination of the newborn directly after birth could prevent this. In Japan, a program was established to screen all pregnant women and, if carriers were found, to make arrangements to vaccinate the newborn. Sensitivity to this problem was required when developing the health-education programs. Mothers often became aware of the serious consequences of the carrier state, which could lead to liver disease and PHC. The knowledge that they might be responsible for passing to their children the causative agent of this potentially deadly disease could be traumatizing if the preventive possibilities were not made patently clear.

There was an additional reason to detect carriers. As already noted and based on extensive research in the United States, Europe, Africa, and Asia starting in the 1970s, it became clear that HBV was the major cause of primary cancer of the liver, which, in many parts of the world, is one of the most common cancers.[12] It is often possible to detect PHC at an early stage before the appearance of any signs or symptoms by the use of a simple blood test that detects alpha fetoprotein (AFP), a protein that is found in the fetus and in newborn children. It is also found in cancers such as PHC which have characteristics of fetal tissues. With the development of the tests for detecting

---

[12] B. S. Blumberg and W. T. London, "Hepatitis B Virus and Prevention of Primary Cancer of the Liver: Guest Editorial," *Journal of the National Cancer Institute* 74 (1985): 267–273.

HBV, high-risk populations could be screened, carriers detected, and then encouraged to attend a prevention center where they could be monitored at regular intervals for any rise in alpha fetoprotein. If an elevated AFP was found, the subject would be admitted for diagnostic imaging designed to detect even small tumors; if any were found, surgery could be performed. Based on clinical experience in China, there was good reason to believe that this early detection and surgery would markedly increase survival.[13]

This represented a second reason for testing the general population for HBV carriers. We established a program at the Fox Chase Cancer Center in Philadelphia, the Liver Cancer Prevention Center, to test the high-risk groups. Hence, the ethical considerations had completely reversed as a consequence of continuing research. Science and ethics are intimately related; scientific discoveries may generate ethical questions, but they can also be used to resolve them.

Research is now in progress which could make it even more beneficial to detect carriers. If it were possible to eliminate the virus from the carriers, this would presumably reduce the risk of developing cancer and also the infectiousness of the carriers. Even if the virus could not be completely removed and the postulated antiviricide were partially effective, it might slow down the process of cell killing and liver dysfunction caused by HBV so that the carrier would remain asymptomatic for a much longer period and live out his or her life expectancy. We have referred to this as "Prevention by Delay."

We are currently investigating a plant-derived medication, which in laboratory and animal studies appears to be effective against HBV.[14] If these studies continue to have encouraging results, and a practical medication is developed, then it might

[13] T. T. Sun and Y. Y. Chu, "Carcinogenesis and Prevention Strategy of Liver Cancer in Areas of Prevalence," *Journal of Cellular Physiology* 3 (1984): 39–44.

[14] P. S. Venkateswaran, I. Millman, and B. S. Blumberg, "Effects of an Extract from *Phylanthus niruri* on Hepatitis B and Woodchuck Hepatitis B Viruses: *In Vitro* and *In Vivo* Studies," *Proceedings of the National Academy of Sciences* 84 (1987): 274–278.

find widespread use for the treatment of carriers. This, in due course, could remove many of the medical and ethical problems related to the carrier state.

* This work was supported by USPHS grants CA-40737, RR-05895 and CA-06927 from the National Institutes of Health and by an appropriation from the Commonwealth of Pennsylvania.

AIDS and Metaphor: Toward the Social Meaning of Epidemic Disease*

BY ALLAN M. BRANDT

No one today need be reminded of the seriousness of the AIDS epidemic. Although much about AIDS remains unclear, it goes without saying that AIDS is a terribly complex and tragic problem; in this first decade of the epidemic, AIDS has already generated untold suffering and an enormous social crisis. Even if we could immediately end all further transmission of the virus, we would be dealing with the disease for decades to come.

The numbers are truly staggering; they provide but a general sense of the full implications of the epidemic. In the United States there have already been more than 100,000 deaths from AIDS; perhaps twice that many individuals are currently in treatment, experiencing a range of symptoms related to infection with the human immunodeficiency virus (HIV). The U.S. Public Health Service projects that more than 1 million individuals are infected with the virus.[1] While the full parameters of the epidemic remain unclear, these figures are nonetheless striking.

The situation in the United States represents but a significant fraction of the worldwide pandemic. The World Health

---

[1] Coolfont Report, Centers for Disease Control, U.S. Public Health Service, 1986.

Organization currently estimates that there are between eight
and 10 million people in the world already infected with HIV.
If projections held true, by the year 2000, 15 million to 20
million will be infected. By that time, 10 million uninfected
children will be orphaned because of the deaths of their mothers and fathers.[2]

Despite swift progress in identifying a causal organism,
biomedical solutions to AIDS appear to be a good way off.
There is currently no curative treatment and no vaccine. As we
now recognize, AIDS constitutes a public-health crisis of global
dimensions, a sad but powerful reminder of our relative
inability to alter the nature of the biological world.

History, Metaphor, and Analogy

What does the history of disease have to tell us about this
epidemic? How can we construct a useful past? These are
recurrent questions as we try to assess the contemporary health
crisis of AIDS. The problem, of course, is not only to find
appropriate and useful analogues, but also to understand the
very process by which diseases have come to be understood—
their particular meaning and significance. History, of course,
holds no simple truths. The historical record is not a fable with
a moral spelled out at the end. Even if we could agree on a
particular construction of past events—and most historians
recognize how difficult this may be—it would not provide a
clear guide to the future. Nevertheless, there are lessons in the
way societies have responded to epidemic disease in the past
that might inform and deepen our understanding of the AIDS
crisis.

Throughout human history, epidemic disease has constituted a natural experiment in how societies respond to
disability, dependence, fear, and death. In this sense, the

[2] *AIDS and the Third World* (Washington, D.C.: Panos Institute, 1986); *New York Times,*
August 2, 1990.

manner in which a society responds reveals its most fundamental cultural, social, and moral values. Disease is not merely a biological phenomenon; it is shaped by powerful behavioral, social, and political forces. Social values affect both the way we come to see and understand a particular disease and the interventions we undertake. In this view, disease is "socially constructed."[3]

Perhaps the most widely read and provocative recent writing on the social meaning of disease is Susan Sontag's *Illness as Metaphor*, first published in the *New York Review of Books* in 1978.[4] Sontag's brilliant polemic was written long before anyone was aware of the human immunodeficiency virus, although it now seems evident that this organism was already silently spreading at that time. Sontag assessed the metaphors typically associated with tuberculosis, the most fearsome disease of nineteenth-century Western societies, and cancer, until recently the most fearsome disease of the twentieth.

"My point," Sontag stated directly, "is that illness is *not* a metaphor, and that the most truthful way of regarding illness—and the healthiest way of being ill—is one most purified of, most resistant to, metaphoric thinking."[5] She argued that metaphors have powerful negative connotations which lead to the isolation and stigmatization of victims of disease. "As long as a particular disease is treated as an evil, invincible predator, not just a disease, most people with cancer will indeed be demoralized by learning what disease they have," wrote Sontag. But what, we might ask, is "just a disease."

[3] For a brief explanation of the "social construction" of disease, see Elliot G. Mishler, *Social Contexts of Health, Illness, and Patient Care* (Cambridge and New York: Cambridge University Press, 1981). For a brilliant historical rendering of the concept, see Charles E. Rosenberg, *The Cholera Years: The United States in 1832, 1849, and 1866* (Chicago: Chicago University Press, 1962; rev. ed. 1987). Rosenberg's account of three major cholera epidemics in New York City remains a classic work in the relationship of disease to social meaning.
[4] Susan Sontag, "Illness as Metaphor," *New York Review of Books* 24 (Jan. 26, 1978); 25 (Feb. 9, 1978); 25 (Feb. 23, 1978).
[5] Susan Sontag, *Illness as Metaphor* (New York: Vintage, 1979), p. 3.

All diseases have particular meanings—meanings that are both historically and culturally specific. These meanings reflect our ability to make sense of the disease scientifically, culturally, and politically; they reflect our notions of the physical and social qualities of the specific disease and its victims.

In at least one critical respect, Sontag missed the mark: disease cannot be freed of metaphors. Despite her plea that illness is *not* a metaphor, the process by which disease acquires meaning and value is ubiquitous. Disease is simply too significant, too basic an aspect of human existence to presume that we could respond in fully rational or neutral ways. Disease raises questions of dependence, debility, and death; it is literally "loaded" with affect and social values. Lethal disease cannot be "demystified" as Sontag would wish. There is no cultural "disinfectant" that is likely to free Western cultures from a deep and profound fear of disabling or lethal disease.[6]

Ultimately, Sontag opts for a notion of positivist science, antiseptic and neutral, that will release us from metaphor, if not disease itself. She posits that with scientific knowledge, the metaphors of disease wither away. In this respect, Sontag misconstrues the significance of modern biological reductionism and the medical search for "magic bullets." Following the guidance of Lewis Thomas, she argues for a theory of monocausality:

> All the diseases for which the issue of causation has been settled, and which can be prevented and cured, have turned out to have a simple physical cause—like the tubercle bacillus for tuberculosis, a single vitamin deficiency for pellagra—and it is far from unlikely that something comparable will eventually be isolated for cancer. The notion that a disease can be explained only by a variety of causes is precisely characteristic of thinking about diseases whose causation is not understood. And it is diseases thought to be multi-determined (that is, mysterious) that have the widest possibilities as metaphors for what is felt to be socially or morally wrong.[7]

[6] See, for example, Philippe Aries, *The Hour of Our Death* (New York: Knopf, 1981). Also, Ernest Becker, *The Denial of Death* (New York: Free Press, 1973).
[7] Sontag, *Illness as Metaphor*, p. 60.

This denies the reality that tuberculosis is, in fact, multicausal. As became clear in the late nineteenth century, after Robert Koch discovered the organism, the tubercle must be present, but it does not *cause* tuberculosis. Moreover, the most dramatic decline in the disease came long before the organism or effective treatments were discovered.[8] Sontag fails to consider that diseases which have many causes—biologic, environmental, social, cultural—may eventually be "solved" through a single intervention. The "magic bullet" does not imply that all diseases ultimately present a unilateral, monolithic target. Moreover, the very nature of the diseases which persist—like heart disease, cancer, syphilis, or AIDS—underscores the variety of forces that cause disease.

Although the "cause" of AIDS is known, the disease is richly metaphorized. Sontag's desire to deny the complex, multicausal aspects of disease betrays a fundamental discomfort with the notion that disease is a social construct. Her positivism denies the emotional cogency of the argument implicit in *Illness as Metaphor*. As her very analysis makes clear, while the meaning of disease is ever changing given our modes of explaining and accounting for the phenomena, illnesses continue to attract the most powerful social and political meanings. Indeed, Sontag derails her very thesis; disease is rife with meaning.

The medical social sciences and humanities offer the potential for deciphering and perhaps bending these meanings. By demonstrating the process by which biology and culture interact, the precise nature of the "social construction" of disease may be revealed. This, of course, is not to argue that disease is a purely relative phenomenon, merely "constructed" by certain privileged knowledge. Rather, it suggests that so complex a phenomenon as disease cannot be understood outside the culture in which it occurs. The biological world is

[8] See Thomas McKeown, *The Role of Medicine* (Princeton: Princeton University Press, 1979).

fundamentally transformed by culture and politics. In this sense, we *use* disease to define social boundaries and psychological stereotypes. Rather than decrying the metaphorization of disease, it seems more appropriate to analyze the process by which disease is given meaning. In this respect, it makes sense to review the history of disease. By drawing careful analogies, recognizing that specific diseases elicit particular responses at historically defined moments, we may come to understand the meaning of disease in our culture at a deeper level.

The Social Construction of Sexually Transmitted Disease

Interestingly enough, Sontag dismissed the metaphors associated with venereal diseases as relatively uninteresting. She suggested that sexually transmitted infections were so thoroughly considered instances of evil that they possessed little significance as metaphors. Nevertheless, the history of sexually transmitted disease in the twentieth century may hold certain lessons for our understanding of the current epidemic.

An examination of the first decades of the twentieth century, a moment of intense concern and interest in sexually transmitted diseases, not unlike those today, may demonstrate how this process has worked. Indeed, the first two decades of the twentieth century witnessed a general hysteria about venereal infections. The historical analogues are striking; they relate to public health, science, and, especially, social and cultural values.

This period, often referred to as the Progressive Era, combined two powerful strains in American social thought: the search for new technical, scientific answers to social problems and the search for a set of unified moral ideals. The problem of sexually transmitted diseases appealed to both sets of interests. The campaign against these infections—the "social hygiene" movement—was predicated on a series of major scientific breakthroughs. The specific organism that causes gonorrhea, the gonococcus, and the causative agent for syphilis, the spirochete, were identified. By the end of the first decade of the twentieth century, diagnostic exams had been established.[9] In 1910, German Nobel laureate Paul Ehrlich discovered the first major chemotherapeutic agent effective against the spirochete. Science had the effect of reframing the way in which these diseases were seen. The enormous social, cultural, and economic costs of venereal disease were finally revealed.

Doctors came to define what they called venereal *insontium,* or venereal disease of the innocent. Victorian physicians traced the tragic repercussions of syphilis within the family. Perhaps the best known example of venereal *insontium* was ophthalmia *neonatorum,* gonorrheal blindness of the newborn. As late as 1910, as many as 25 percent of all the blind in the United States had lost their sight in this way, despite the earlier discovery that silver-nitrate solution could prevent infection. Soon many states began to require the use of the prophylactic treatment by law.[10]

But doctors stressed the impact on women even more than children. In 1906 the AMA held a symposium on "The Duty of the Profession to Womanhood." As one physician at the conference explained:

These vipers of venery which are called clap and pox, lurking as they often do, under the floral tributes of the honeymoon, may

---

[9] The following discussion is abbreviated from my book *No Magic Bullet: A Social History of Venereal Disease in the United States since 1880* (New York: Oxford University Press, 1985; rev. ed., 1987).

[10] On the problem of ophthalmia *neonatorum,* see Abraham L. Wolbarst, "On the Occurrence of Syphilis and Gonorrhea in Children by Direct Infection," *American Medicine* 7 (1912): 494; Carolyn Von Blarcum, "The Harm Done in Ascribing All Babies' Sore Eyes to Gonorrhea," *American Journal of Public Health* 6 (1916): 926–931; and J.W. Kerr, "Ophthalmia neonatorum: An Analysis of the Laws and Regulations in Relation thereto in Force in the United States," *Public Health Service Bulletin,* no. 49 (Washington, D.C., 1914).

so inhibit conception or blight its products that motherhood becomes either an utter impossibility or a veritable curse. The ban placed by venereal disease on fetal life outrivals the criminal interference with the products of conception as a cause of race suicide.[11]

The train of family tragedy was a frequent cultural theme in these years. In 1913 a hit Broadway play by French playwright Eugene Brieux, *Damaged Goods,* told the story of young George Dupont, who, though warned by his physician not to marry because he has syphilis, disregards this advice only to spread the infection to his wife and, later, to their child. This story was told and retold, and it revealed deep cultural values about science, social responsibility, and the limits of medicine to cure the moral ailments of humankind.[12]

But physicians expressed concerns that went beyond the confines of the family; they also examined the wider social repercussions of sexually transmitted diseases. The last years of the nineteenth century and the first of the twentieth were the most intensive periods of immigration to the United States in its entire history; more than 650,000 immigrants came to these shores each year between 1885 and 1910. Many doctors and social critics suggested that these individuals were bringing venereal disease into the country. As Howard Kelly, a leading gynecologist at Johns Hopkins, explained, "The tide [of venereal disease] has been raising [sic] owing to the inpouring of a large foreign population with lower ideals." Kelly elaborated, warning, "Think of these countless currents flowing daily from the houses of the poorest into those of the

---

[11] Albert H. Burr, "The Guarantee of Safety in the Marriage Contract," *Journal of the American Medical Association* 47 (1906): 1887–88.

[12] See Eugene Brieux, *Damaged Goods,* tr. John Pollack (New York: Brentano's, 1913). On the critical reception of the play, see "Demoralizing Plays," *Outlook* 150 (1913): 110; John D. Rockefeller, "The Awakening of a New Social Conscience," *Medical Reviews of Reviews* 19 (1913): 281; "Damaged Goods," *Hearst's Magazine* 23 (1913): 806; "Brieux's New Sociological Sermon in Three Acts," *Current Opinion* 54 (1913): 296–297.

See also Barbara Gutmann Rosenkrantz, "Damaged Goods: Dilemmas of Responsibility for Risk," *Milbank Memorial Fund Quarterly* 57 (1979): 1–37.

richest, and forming a sort of civic circulatory system expressive of the body politic, a circulation which continually tends to equalize the distribution of morality and disease."[13]

Examinations at the ports of entry failed to reveal a high incidence of disease. Nevertheless, nativists called for the restriction of immigration. How were these immigrants spreading sexually transmitted diseases to native, middle-class, Anglo-Saxon Americans? First, it was suggested that immigrants constituted the great bulk of the prostitutes who inhabited American cities; virtually every major American metropolis of the early twentieth century had defined red-light districts where prostitution flourished. These women, it was suggested, were typically foreign born.[14]

But even more importantly, physicians now asserted that syphilis and gonorrhea could be transmitted in any number of ways. Doctors catalogued the various modes of transmission. Pens, pencils, toothbrushes, towels and bedding, and medical procedures were all identified as potential means of communication.[15] As one woman explained in an anonymous essay in 1912:

> At first it was unbelievable. I knew of the disease only through newspaper advertisements [for patent medicines]. I had understood that it was the result of sin and that it originated and was contracted only in the underworld of the city. I felt sure that my friend was mistaken in diagnosis when he exclaimed, "Another tragedy of the common drinking cup!" I eagerly met his remark with the assurance that I did not use public drinking cups, that I had used my own cup for years. He led me to review my

[13] Howard Kelly, "Social Diseases and Their Prevention," *Social Diseases* 1 (1910): 17; idem, "The Protection of the Innocent," *American Journal of Obstetrics* 55 (1907): 477–481.

[14] On prostitution in Progressive America, see Paul S. Boyer, *Urban Masses and Moral Order* (Cambridge: Harvard University Press, 1978); Ruth Rosen, *The Lost Sisterhood: Prostitution on America, 1900–1918* (Baltimore: Johns Hopkins University Press, 1982); and Mark Thomas Connelly, *The Response to Prostitution in the Progressive Era* (Chapel Hill: University of North Carolina Press, 1980).

[15] On nonvenereal transmission, see especially L. Duncan Bulkey, *Syphilis of the Innocent* (New York: Bailey & Fairchild, 1894).

summer. After recalling a number of times when my thirst had
forced me to go to the public fountain, I came at last to realize
that what he had told me was true.[16]

The doctor, of course, had diagnosed syphilis. One indication
of how seriously these casual modes of transmission were taken
is the fact that the Navy removed doorknobs from its
battleships during the First World War, claiming that they had
been a source of infection for many of its sailors (a remarkable
act of denial). We now know, of course, that syphilis and
gonorrhea cannot be contracted in these ways. This poses a
difficult historical problem: why did physicians believe that
they could be?

Theories of casual transmission reflected deep cultural fears
about disease and sexuality in the early twentieth century. In
these approaches to venereal disease, concerns about hygiene,
contamination, and contagion were expressed, anxieties that
reflected a great deal about the contemporary society and
culture. Venereal disease was viewed as a threat to the entire
late Victorian social and sexual system, which placed great
value on discipline, restraint, and homogeneity. The sexual
code of this era held that only sex-in-marriage should receive
social sanction. But the concerns about venereal disease also
reflected a pervasive fear of the urban masses, the growth of
the cities, and the changing nature of familial relationships.
Finally, the distinction between venereal disease and venereal
insontium had the effect of dividing victims; some deserved
attention, sympathy, and medical support, others did not.
This, of course, depended on how the infection was obtained.
Victims were separated into the innocent and the guilty.

In short, venereal disease became a metaphor for the
anxieties of this time, reflecting deep social and cultural values
about sexuality, contagion, and social organization. But these
metaphors are not simply innocuous linguistic constructions.

---

[16] "What One Woman Has Had to Bear," *Forum* 68 (1912): 451–454. See also "New
Laws About Drinking Cups," *Life* 58 (1911): 1152.

They have powerful sociopolitical implications, many of which have been remarkably persistent during the twentieth century.

These concerns about sexually transmitted diseases led to a major public-health campaign to stop their spread. Many of the public-health approaches that we apply today to communicable infections were developed in the early years of the twentieth century. Educational programs formed a major component of the campaign. But to speak of education is far too vague. The question, of course, is the precise content of the education offered. During the first decades of the twentieth century, when schools first instituted sex-education programs, their basic goal was to encourage premarital continence by inculcating fear of sex. Indeed, it would be more accurate to call these programs antisex education.

The new ability to diagnose syphilis and gonorrhea led to the development of other important public-health interventions. Indeed, most of the public-health interventions that we associate with communicable diseases were established in the early years of the twentieth century in response to sexually transmitted diseases. Reporting, screening, testing, and isolation of carriers were all initiated as venereal-disease-control measures. American cities began to require the reporting of venereal diseases around 1915. Some states used reports to follow contacts and bring individuals in for treatment. By the 1930s many states had come to require premarital and prenatal screening. Some municipalities mandated compulsory screening of food handlers and barbers, even though it was by then understood that syphilis and gonorrhea could not be spread through casual contact. The rationale offered was that these individuals were at risk for infection anyway and that screening might reveal new cases for treatment.

Perhaps the most dramatic public-health intervention devised to combat sexually transmitted diseases was the campaign to close red-light districts. In the first two decades of the twentieth century, vice commissions in almost all American cities identified prostitutes as a major risk for American health and morals and decided that the time had come to remove the sources of infection. Comparing the red-light districts to malaria-producing swamps, they attempted to "drain" these swamps. During the First World War more than a hundred red-light districts were closed. The crackdown on prostitutes constituted the most concerted attack on civil liberties in the name of public health in American history. Not surprisingly, in the atmosphere of crisis that the war engendered, public-health officials employed radical techniques in their battle against venereal disease. State laws held that anyone "reasonably suspected" of harboring a venereal infection could be tested on a compulsory basis. Prostitutes were now subject to quarantine, detention, and internment.[17] Attorney General T. W. Gregory explained:

> The constitutional right of the community, in the interest of the public health, to ascertain the existence of infection and communicable diseases in its midst and to isolate and quarantine such cases or take steps necessary to prevent the spread of disease is clear.[18]

In July 1918, Congress allocated more than $1 million for the detention and isolation of venereal carriers. During the war more than 30,000 prostitutes were incarcerated in institutions supported by the federal government. As one federal official noted:

> Conditions required the immediate isolation of as many venereally infected persons acting as spreaders of disease as

[17] The wartime policy for the attack on the red-light districts and the testing and incarceration of prostitutes is described in greater detail in Brandt, *No Magic Bullet*, pp. 80–95.

[18] T. W. Gregory, "Memorandum on Legal Aspects of the Proposed System of Medical Examination of Women Convicted Under Section 13, Selective Service Act," National Archives, Washington, D.C., Record Group 90, Box 223. See Also Mary Macey Dietzler, *Detention Houses and Reformatories as Protective Social Agencies in the Campaign of the United States Government Against Venereal Diseases*, United States Interdepartmental Social Hygiene Board (Washington: Government Printing Office, 1922).

could be quickly apprehended and quarantined. It was not a measure instituted for the punishment of prostitutes on account of infraction of the civil or moral law, but was strictly a public health measure to prevent the spread of dangerous, communicable diseases.[19]

Fear of venereal disease during the war had led to substantial inroads against traditional civil liberties. Although many of these interventions were challenged in the courts, most were upheld; the police powers of the state were deemed sufficient to override any constitutional concerns. The program of detention and isolation, it should be noted, had no impact on rates of venereal disease, which increased dramatically during the war. Although this story is not well known, it is not unlike the internment of Japanese-Americans during World War II.

AIDS in a Cultural Context

In light of the history of sexually transmitted diseases in the last century, it is almost impossible to watch the AIDS epidemic without experiencing a sense of déjà vu. AIDS raises a host of concerns traditional to the debates about venereal infection, from morality to medicine, sexuality and deviancy, prevention and intervention. In many instances the situation with AIDS today is similar to that with syphilis in the early twentieth century. As with syphilis, AIDS can cause death; currently has no curative treatment; is being attacked by means of education and social engineering given that no magic bullet is on the horizon; and arouses fears that reflect deeper social and cultural anxieties about the disease, its transmissibility, and its victims. And yet AIDS is different.

AIDS has threatened our sense of medical security. After all,

[19] C. C. Pierce, "The Value of Detention as a Reconstruction Measure," *American Journal of Obstetrics* 80 (1919): 629.

the age of transmissible, lethal infections was deemed long past in the Western world. Ours was the age of chronic disease— heart diseases and cancers that principally strike late in life. Communicability—epidemics of infectious diseases—had receded in the public memory. Not since the polio epidemics of the 1950s has fear of infection reached such a high pitch as it has in the 1980s. Indeed, no epidemic since the swine flu pandemic of 1918 has had such a dramatic impact on patterns of mortality. And ironically, the concerns in 1976 about a new epidemic of swine flu, which never materialized, seemed to confirm that fear of epidemic infection was unfounded in this modern age of antibiotics. AIDS has fractured this false sense of confidence. Effective responses to such a problem are further complicated by its "social construction," those attitudes and values that shape the public view of the disease. The social construction of AIDS will in turn have a powerful impact on the choices made in responding to the disease.

A number of factors in the way in which AIDS is "defined" greatly complicate the development of appropriate social policies. Among the most prominent is the context of fear and uncertainty that characterize the epidemic. Despite considerable progress in the scientific and medical understanding of AIDS, much remains unknown. Given the lethal dangers of infection, concerns have remained high and the public is not easily reassured about the risks. Postwar American culture has little experience tolerating the uncertainties of epidemic disease. Moreover, the epidemic has arrived during an era of decline in the authority of experts.[20] Three Mile Island, Chernobyl, and the disaster of the space shuttle have encouraged public distrust of official reassurances that catastrophe cannot happen.

Given a fall in the legitimacy of experts, the social process of

[20] Leon Eisenberg, "Private Trust/Public Confidence in Science and Medicine: The Genesis of Fear," *Law Medicine and Health Care* 14 (1986): 243–249; Robert Balzell, "The History of an Epidemic," *New Republic* 189 (Aug. 1, 1983): 14–18; Richard Goldstein, "The Uses of AIDS," *Village Voice*, Nov. 5, 1985, pp. 25–27.

evaluating relative risks becomes difficult. In 1985, parents in Queens, New York, called for a boycott of public schools because an HIV-infected student was permitted to attend. Their concerns could not be mollified in light of the persistent uncertainties about the disease. As a culture, our relative lack of sophistication in comparing risks has been exacerbated by the fear of AIDS.[21] One angry parent reportedly told a public-health official, "You send my child home when he has head lice. Now you want me to send my child to school with another child who has an infection which you just said is always fatal." The epidemic raises serious questions about the nature of risk assessment, scientific literacy, and counterintuitive reasoning. All of which suggests the need for better public education at all levels.

The risks of AIDS have also been difficult to calibrate in the political arena. As a political culture we tend to reject policies when their costs become clear—even if they may offer significant benefits. While all social policies carry some costs, we have tended to seek those policies that appear to be cost-free. Take, for example, the debate concerning the provision of sterile needles for intravenous drug users. Such programs have been proposed as one possible measure for controlling the spread of infection. Nevertheless, proposals have drawn powerful criticism principally because of the concern that the provision of needles will be viewed as officially sanctioning and encouraging drug abuse. In this respect, the costs of a potentially beneficial program are viewed as too high. The same could be said for explicit education to encourage safer sexual behavior. The federal government has rejected support of such efforts, fearing that support will be politically perceived as an endorsement of homosexuality or teenage premarital sex. There is more than

[21] "The Fear of AIDS," *Newsweek* 106 (Sept. 23, 1985): 18–25. On the school controversy, see *New York Times*, Oct. 13, 24, 1985, Dec. 8, 1985. Also David J. Rothman, "Public Policy and Risk Assessment in the Case of AIDS," in *AIDS: Public Policy Dimensions* (New York: United Hospital Fund, 1986).

hypocrisy behind the opposition to such programs; there are powerful presumptions that the disease itself must be *used* to discourage risky behaviors.

On the other hand, policies which offer little in relation to public health often have considerable appeal. "Better safe than sorry" logic could lead to compulsory interventions that fundamentally compromise civil liberties yet offer little potential benefit. The pressure to "do something" could well result in useless and ultimately destructive policies. For example, Illinois and Louisiana recently enacted provisions for compulsory premarital screening for HIV, and similar laws are under consideration in many states. Such programs are unlikely to find many new, unknown cases of infection because they are directed at individuals unlikely to have been at principal risk for infection. Therefore, they are likely to find large numbers of false positives.[22] Moreover, such programs are costly and deflect funding from programs more likely to have an impact on the epidemic.

The fact that the two principal high-risk groups are already highly stigmatized in American culture has had a powerful impact on responses to the epidemic. Some have seen the AIDS epidemic in a purely "moral" light: AIDS is a disease that occurs among those who violate the moral order. As one journalist concluded: "Suddenly a lot of people fear that they and their families might suddenly catch some mysterious, fatal illness which until now has been confined to society's social outcasts." AIDS, like other sexually transmitted diseases in the past, has been viewed as a fateful link between social deviance and the morally correct. Such fears have been exacerbated by an expectant media. "NO ONE IS SAFE FROM AIDS," announced *Life* in bold red letters on its cover.[23] Implicit was the notion that "no one is safe" from gays and intravenous

---

[22] See, for example, P. Cleary and others, "Compulsory Screening for the Human Immunodeficiency Virus," *Journal of the American Medical Association* 258 (1987): 1757–62.

[23] *Life* 8 (July 1985): 12–21.

drug abusers. The disease had come to be equated with those who are at highest risk of suffering its terrible consequences.

Underlying the fears of transmission were deeper concerns about homosexuality. Just as "innocent syphilis" in the first decades of the twentieth century was thought to bring the "respectable middle-class" in contact with a deviant, ethnic, working-class "sexual underworld," now AIDS threatened the heterosexual culture with homosexual contamination. In this context, homosexuality—not a virus—*causes* AIDS. Therefore, homosexuality itself is feared as if it were a communicable, lethal disease. After a generation of work to have homosexuality removed as a disease from the psychiatric diagnostic manuals, it had suddenly reappeared as an infectious, terminal disease.[24]

The AIDS epidemic thus offered new opportunities for the expression of moral opprobrium for homosexuality. Patrick Buchanan, conservative columnist and former Reagan speechwriter, explained, "The poor homosexuals—they have declared war upon Nature, and now Nature is exacting an awful retribution."[25] Criticizing government expenditures on research to produce a vaccine, editor Norman Podhoretz wrote, "Are they aware that in the name of compassion they are giving social sanction to what can only be described as brutish degradation?"[26] Podhoretz's position—that gays get what they deserve, that to investigate treatments would merely encourage unhealthy behaviors—is a characteristic position in the history of sexually transmitted diseases. It also indicates a remarkably uninformed view of the epidemic, as well as a complete disregard for the public health.

How can victim-blaming and stigmatization of high-risk, already socially outcast groups be avoided? In many respects the process of dividing victims into blameless and blameful—

---

[24] See Ronald Bayer, *Homosexuality and American Psychiatry: The Politics of Diagnosis* (New York: Basic Books, 1981).

[25] *New York Post,* May 24, 1983.

[26] Quoted in *New York Times,* Mar. 18, 1986.

analogous to early-twentieth-century notions of venereal disease *insontium*—has been activated once again. This can be seen, for example, in assessments such as the following offered by a journalist in the *New York Times Magazine* in 1983:

> The groups most recently found to be at risk for AIDS present a particularly poignant problem. Innocent bystanders caught in the path of a new disease, they can make no behavioral decisions to minimize their risk: hemophiliacs cannot stop taking bloodclotting medication; surgery patients cannot stop getting transfusions; women cannot control the drug habits of their mates; babies cannot choose their mothers.[27]

This passage raises a number of problems. First, it suggests that the disease is somehow more "poignant" when it attacks nonhomosexuals. Second, if these groups are "innocent bystanders," then those at highest risk of contracting AIDS may be assumed to be "guilty." Implicit in this discussion is the view that the entire community is at risk from the sexual practices of homosexuals. In some quarters the misapprehension persists: AIDS is caused by homosexuality rather than by a retrovirus. In this confused logic, the answer to the problem is simple: repress these behaviors. Implicit in this approach to the problem are powerful notions of culpability and guilt.[28]

Such themes are contained in the metaphors of the AIDS epidemic. A number of health educators, including Surgeon General C. Everett Koop, recently told audiences, "When you have sex with someone you're really having sex with all of their partners for perhaps as long as the last ten years." This is a metaphor with a range of meanings. At a moment when the dangers of promiscuous sex are being emphasized, it suggests every *single* sexual encounter is a promiscuous encounter; an individual may well be having intercourse with *many* partners.

[27] Robin Marantz Henig, "AIDS: A New Disease's Deadly Odyssey," *New York Times Magazine,* Feb. 6, 1983, p. 36.

[28] See, for example, John H. Knowles, "The Responsibility of the Individual," *Daedalus* 106 (1977): 68; and Robert Carlen, "Against Free Clinics for Sexually Transmitted Diseases," *New England Journal of Medicine* 307 (1982): 1350.

As anonymous sex is being questioned, this metaphor suggests that no matter how well known a partner may be, the relationship is *anonymous*. Finally, the metaphor implies to heterosexuals that if they are having sex with their partner's (heterosexual) partners, they are in fact engaging in homosexual acts. In this view, every sexual act becomes a homosexual encounter. Obviously, I do not want to suggest that Koop intends to make these suggestions when he recites this metaphor. The very nature of metaphor is that it works on many levels, conscious and unconscious, explicit and implicit. Its meanings are typically hidden in the culture. No one could suggest, however, that this metaphor does not intend to invoke fear of sex. Implicit in such metaphors is the idea of making sexuality itself deviant.

Assessments of AIDS—as of most sexually transmitted diseases in the twentieth century—rest on the essentially simplistic view that the problem can be solved if individuals conduct their sexual lives more responsibly. The assumption that an individual's behavior is free from external forces—that lifestyle is strictly voluntary—is explicit. These persistent assumptions about health-related behavior rest upon an essentially naive, simplistic view of human nature. If anything has become clear in the course of the twentieth century it is that behavior is subject to complex forces, internal psychologies and external pressures, all of which are not subject to immediate modification or, arguably, to modification at all. Sexuality is subject to a number of powerful influences, social and economic, conscious and unconscious, many more powerful than even the fear of disease. "Just Say No" will not end the epidemic of drug abuse or the AIDS epidemic.

A generation from now historians may look back at the AIDS epidemic, proud of our capacity to forthrightly and humanely address a profound human crisis—or they may look back marking AIDS as the crisis that fundamentally exacerbated the bitterest divisions of our society. The social costs of ineffective, draconian public-health measures would only augment the crisis we know as AIDS. But such measures can be avoided only if we are adept in both our medical and cultural understanding of this disease and its metaphors. For we need to perform a difficult task, that of separating deeply irrational fears from scientific understanding. Only when we recognize the ways in which social and cultural values shape this disease will we be able to begin to deal justly, humanely, and effectively with a problem as serious and complex as AIDS.

* Portions of this essay are drawn from my book *No Magic Bullet: A Social History of Venereal Disease in the United States since 1880* (New York: Oxford University Press, 1985; rev. ed., 1987).

Responses to Plague in Early Modern Europe: The Implications of Public Health

BY PAUL SLACK

Bᴇᴛᴡᴇᴇɴ the Black Death of the fourteenth century and the great epidemics in Marseilles and Moscow in the eighteenth century, bubonic plague was responsible for a succession of the greatest epidemic disasters in recorded history. That is one reason why any symposium on past and present pestilences ought to consider it. Another is that these outbreaks of plague, extending over four centuries, elicited positive social responses. They stimulated deliberate defensive measures which were socially formative and profoundly controversial at the time, and which have shaped the concepts and practices of "public health" ever since.

It was during epidemics of bubonic plague that the towns of late medieval and early modern Europe first developed sophisticated mechanisms intended to control the spread of epidemic disease and to mitigate its effects. Plague victims were isolated and their contacts traced and incarcerated. There were restrictions on movement, bills of health, quarantine regulations for travelers and shipping. Bedding and houses were fumigated. All this necessitated the growth of local administrative machines and an expansion of state power, the invention of "medical police" in fact. It also implied serious restrictions on individual liberty and provoked opposition for that reason, among others. Those conflicts between public and private interests and between the dictates of medically informed prudence and the imperatives of popular morality, which arose in the case of later epidemics from cholera to AIDS, can first be fully documented in Europe in the age of plague.

The critical nature of the phenomenon to which early modern Europeans had to respond can be summarized very briefly. The mortality levels reached during outbreaks of plague were unparalleled. During the Black Death itself, between 1347 and 1351, it is estimated that something like a third of the population of Europe died. Bubonic plague never again caused that level of fatality over whole countries, but it continued to levy death tolls of similar proportions in individual towns and cities. In Venice in 1347–48 and Genoa in 1656–57, 60 percent of the population is estimated to have died; half the population of Milan died in an outbreak of plague in 1630, and perhaps half the population of Padua in 1405 and of Lyons in 1628–29; the death toll reached 30 percent or more in Norwich, England, in 1579, in Venice in 1630–31, in Marseilles in 1720, and in Moscow in 1771.[1] Furthermore, mortalities of this kind were achieved in a very short space of time, usually within six months, between June and December. There can be no question about the scale of the crises caused by plague.

These great and sudden disasters cannot wholly account for the developed response to plague in early modern Europe, however; for there was plainly little opportunity to do more

[1] R. S. Gottfried, *The Black Death* (New York, 1983), p. 48; C. M. Cipolla, *Fighting the Plague in Seventeenth-Century Italy* (Madison, 1981), p. 100; J. N. Biraben, *Les hommes et la peste en France et dans les pays européens et méditerranéans* (Paris, 1975–76), 1: 186, 189, 308; C. M. Cipolla, *Cristofano and the Plague* (London, 1973), p. 20; P. Slack, *The Impact of Plague in Tudor and Stuart England* (London, 1985), pp. 129–30; J. T. Alexander, *Bubonic Plague in Early Modern Russia* (Baltimore, 1980), p. 260.

than flee from them, if one could. There are other features of plague which are equally important in shaping the social response. First, there is the fact that plague recurred again and again in the same places, over centuries. In London, for example, there were at least seventeen outbreaks of plague between 1500 and the last outbreak—the so-called "Great Plague of London"—in 1665. Second, several of these epidemics were of comparatively modest dimensions; and they thus gave people an opportunity to observe the disease in operation more coolly than they could in major crises. The death rate was probably less than 12 percent in the majority of the outbreaks in London, and it is in these relatively minor epidemics, in London and elsewhere, that we find most evidence of contemporaries deliberately planning administrative responses.[2]

Third, and finally, there were features of plague which seemed regular and predictable, as it was observed over the years, in motion across continents and countries, traveling from one place to another. No one knew precisely how it moved. The etiology and epidemiology of plague were not worked out until the end of the nineteenth century. The role of rats and fleas as carriers of the disease was not yet appreciated. There were also puzzling features in the spread of plague. It missed some towns in its transit along major highways, some houses in its movement along a street, some individuals in its progress through a household. Yet it did move in what were, in the end, predictable directions: from ports to other cities, from cities to surrounding villages, from one house to another. In short, plague embodied in a perhaps extreme degree that combination of the predictable and the unpredictable which characterizes all epidemic diseases; and it was this combination—of frequent occurrence but irregular timing, of sometimes high and sometimes low mortality, of

[2] Slack, *Impact of Plague*, pp. 61–62, 206; A. G. Carmichael, *Plague and the Poor in Renaissance Florence* (Cambridge, 1986), p. 107.

movement from person to person and town to town in haphazard ways—which meant that contemporaries both had to develop responses to it and were uncertain and divided over what those responses should be.

The Interpretative System

It is not surprising, in Christian Europe, that so severe and unpredictable a disease should be accorded a supernatural origin. Plague was a divine scourge, a retribution for the sins of mankind: sometimes for sins in general, more often for the specific misdeeds of the time or place of an epidemic. It was God's punishment for new-fangled women's fashions, for swearing and drunkenness, for heresy or atheism, for Protestantism or Catholicism, depending on which side you were on. Repentance and prayer were therefore universally recognized as the proper and first recourse against an epidemic of plague, and these were demonstrated publicly as well as privately, in processions in Catholic countries for most of the period, in public fasts and sermons in Protestant countries after the Reformation.[3] The battle against sin could also be waged against specific targets, by means, for example, of the sumptuary regulations and measures to reform popular manners which were sometimes elements in the response of civic magistrates to plague.[4]

If divine providence came first, however, it worked its purposes through natural causes, which could be understood and against which God had provided medicines and precau-

[3] E.g., B. Bennassar, *Recherches sur les grandes épidémies dans le nord de l'Espagne á la fin du XVIe siècle* (Paris, 1969), p. 55; G. Calvi, "A Metaphor for Social Exchange: The Florentine Plague of 1630," *Representations* 13 (1986): 140; E. Carpentier, *Une ville devant la peste: Orvieto et la peste noire de 1348* (Paris, 1962), p. 155; Slack, *Impact of Plague*, p. 229. For the role of providence more generally in perception of disease, see K. Thomas, *Religion and the Decline of Magic* (London, 1971), ch. 4.

[4] E.g., S. Schama, *The Embarrassment of Riches* (London, 1987), p. 336; Bennassar, *Recherches*, pp. 26, 55.

tions which he intended men to use. The natural causes of plague were many—from disorders in the heavens to earthquakes and unburied corpses—but they all produced "miasma," the bad air of an infected place. This was the immediate cause of disease. It clung to infected towns, as disease did, and it could be attacked there by fumigants and perfumes of various kinds, by setting off guns or lighting bonfires in the streets, as in London in the sixteenth and seventeenth centuries.[5] But miasma could also be transported—in the clothes, bedding, baggage of infected people, or on their persons. It could be picked up from the proximity of the sick and absorbed through the pores of the healthy. Theories of miasma and concepts of contagion were thus combined. The disease could be transmitted from place to place and person to person, and that obviously had repercussions for action. The sick and anything connected with them should be avoided.

There was one final element in contemporary views of plague, as they were articulated in the first plague tractates of the later Middle Ages and transmitted in popular medical manuals down to the eighteenth century.[6] It was necessary to explain why, in an infected place, suffused by miasma, with the danger of contagion all around, some people succumbed to plague and others did not. The answer lay in predisposing causes. Individuals could be temperamentally prone to plague because of an imbalance in their humors. But they also made themselves vulnerable by the abuse of God's gifts, by neglecting the golden mean in their behavior, by too little or (more often) too much food, drink, exercise, emotion, or sexual activity. Here the explanatory wheel came full circle. For these excesses were sinful as well as unhealthy, morally as well as physically dangerous; and the two qualities were

[5] F. P. Wilson, *The Plague in Shakespeare's London* (Oxford, 1963), pp. 31, 169; J. Delumeau, *La Peur en Occident* (Paris, 1978), p. 103; E. Woehlkens, *Pest und Ruhr im 16. und 17. Jahrhundert* (Hanover, 1954), p. 27.
[6] Cf. A. M. Campbell, *The Black Death and Men of Learning* (New York, 1931), ch. 3.

inseparable. The corruption which lay at the root of plague was not only a physical process but also a moral one. There were thus several facets to the concepts of "dis-ease," "disorder," "corruption," and "putrefaction" which contemporaries used to interpret plague; and these evocative terms echo through all the plague literature of early modern Europe, determining the ways in which the pestilence and its victims were regarded.

There are two general points worth stressing here. The first is the essential coherence of this interpretative system. It certainly contained inconsistencies within it, and these were sometimes brought to the surface when writers gave special emphasis to one element at the expense of others. A stress on contagion might seem to involve a denial of the importance of miasma, for example; and the precautionary measures of governments were sometimes taken to imply a rejection of the role of providence. But these tensions were generally suppressed with some success. The explanatory circle held together into the age of cholera. The second point of interest is the way in which this set of assumptions and arguments impelled public actions, in spite of—or perhaps because of—its acknowledgment of the prime role of providence. It is instructive here to compare Christian Europe with the Islamic world. In Moslem countries there was real fatalism in the face of plague: epidemic disease was regarded as a mercy sent by God, which should be welcomed, not combated. No effort was made to take precautions against it or to isolate its victims. In the Christian tradition, by contrast, plague was a punishment, which ought not to have been necessary, for sins which should be identified and rooted out. The Christian view therefore predisposed men to action of various kinds: a search for scapegoats, certainly, a condemnation of the infected, especially if they were poor or otherwise disreputable, but also the elimination of conditions which threatened moral and physical health: large and disorderly public assemblies, for example, or the unruly taverns and alehouses and dirty slums which were the haunts of beggars and vagrants. Moral and social prejudices were a fundamental part—and not by any means always a wholly negative or unproductive part—of public responses to plague.[7]

Plague was thus made consistent with the intellectual presuppositions, the frame of mind, of early modern Europeans; and that enabled them to come to terms with it, to see it in proportion, as it were, as part of a providential order of things. The exceptional stresses which major epidemics imposed on individuals, families, and whole communities should not, of course, be underrated. But there was in fact much less blind panic in plague-time than some popular writers and even some historians have supposed. There was some rationale to most reactions to plague, whether private, popular, or public; there was surprisingly little in the way of simple crowd hysteria or individual psychopathology. Most books on the Black Death describe the bands of flagellants who wandered over much of Europe, scourging themselves, and the attacks on Jews, who were widely treated as scapegoats in that same initial disaster. But both reactions had precedents in the past and were reflections of the contemporary assumptions, first, that plague was punishment for sin and, second, that it was brought into a community by outsiders.[8] These extravagant phenomena were absent from later epidemics, though foreigners and witches were occasionally blamed for an outbreak. There were stories also of men deliberately spreading plague and rumors that people had been buried alive or murdered by their nurses.[9] But much of this was sensational gossip, with little basis in fact.

[7] M. W. Dols, *The Black Death in the Middle East* (Princeton, 1977), pp. 285–298; Slack, *Impact of Plague*, pp. 49–50.

[8] Gottfried, *Black Death*, pp. 69, 73–74; Biraben, *Les hommes et la peste*, 1: 65–71; Delumeau, *La peur*, pp. 132–133. It seems to me that Delumeau greatly exaggerates the collective panic caused by bubonic plague.

[9] Delumeau, *La peur*, pp. 133–134; Calvi, "Metaphor for Social Exchange," pp. 148–151; Slack, *Impact of Plague*, pp. 274–275, 293, 301.

Public Authority

Much more common were two more pedestrian responses: first, flight from infected towns—a sensible precaution, and one which was recommended by most medical writers as the only sure preservative; and second, a hard-headed and sometimes ruthless care for the preservation of self and family even if that meant cruelty to more distant relations, dependents, or neighbors. Servants were turned out into the streets by their masters if they caught plague. Neighbors sometimes refused charitable help to one another, and the infected were denied a decent burial, so that they often had to be interred in their own gardens.[10] Again, however, these were perfectly comprehensible reactions to infectious disease: as one sixteenth-century theologian recognized, in a plague "that which is not so near must give place to the nearer."[11] In these circumstances, what is remarkable is not how often people resorted to *sauve qui peut* as a behavioral maxim but how frequently they ignored prudential precautions in order to help their friends and neighbors. As a result, the social supports of family and neighborhood were rarely demolished completely, even in the greatest disasters. More important for our purposes is the fact that structures of government were also maintained. Magistrates and councillors, those in public authority, generally remained in an infected town, or a sufficient number of them did so. They had sent away wives and children first. They stayed in greater numbers in minor epidemics than in major ones, and they observed the progress of plague more closely and fought it more tenaciously then.[12] But as time went on, they developed a policy for public health which testified to their dedication to strict government and public order even at some personal risk to themselves.

[10] *Ibid.*, pp. 79, 166–169, 288–289; Campbell, *Black Death*, p. 92; Delumeau, *La peur*, pp. 121, 126–127; Biraben, *Les hommes et la peste*, 2: 168–169.

[11] Slack, *Impact of Plague*, p. 290.

[12] *Ibid.*, pp. 257–266.

The first reaction of civic governments to outbreaks of plague at home was, nevertheless, a studied refusal to contemplate them, or at least a denial of their existence for as long as possible.[13] This was as much a matter of policy as of wishful thinking. Public acknowledgment of an epidemic meant the spontaneous flight of the richer inhabitants and immediate damage to commerce, when magistrates elsewhere took protective action. For the chief concern of all municipalities was to prevent plague arriving in the first place. Bans on the movement of goods and people from infected towns began in 1348 and became ever more sophisticated in the following centuries. An infected city found itself ostracized and was granted help from outside only on condition that it maintained itself in isolation. In the seventeenth century the magistrates of English counties arranged the provision of food for infected towns, provided that no one wandered out of them. By the eighteenth century *cordons sanitaires* around plague-stricken cities were common, often maintained by military force, as in the case of Marseilles in 1720.[14] Whatever their consequences for the infected communities themselves—and these were obviously very grave—there is considerable evidence that these measures could be effective in limiting the transmission of plague across space.[15]

Still more effective, certainly in the longer term, was control of shipping by means of bills of health and quarantine stations. That began in the fifteenth century, and by the seventeenth century ports in southern Europe were cooperating with one

[13] *Ibid.*, pp. 256–257; Delumeau, *La peur*, pp. 108–109; Bennassar, *Recherches*, pp. 56–57; E. Rodenwaldt, *Pest in Venedig 1575–1577* (Heidelberg, 1953), p. 41. Cf. C. M. Cipolla, *Public Health and the Medical Profession in the Renaissance* (Cambridge, 1976), p. 53.

[14] Carmichael, *Plague and the Poor*, pp. 99, 115–18; Slack, *Impact of Plague*, pp. 266–268; Biraben, *Les hommes et la peste*, 1: 245–251, 2: 88.

[15] Slack, *Impact of Plague*, pp. 315–321. For other examples, both of success and failure in such controls, see Alexander, *Bubonic Plague and Russia*, pp. 20, 33–35; J. Revel, "Autour d'une épidémie ancienne: La peste de 1666–70," *Revue d'histoire moderne et contemporaine* 17 (1970): 971–973.

another to monitor the movement of suspect ships from the Levant, the usual source of new waves of infection.[16] The failure of such measures in Marseilles in 1720 led to the great epidemic there, but that is arguably the exception which proves the rule that controls on shipping might in the end limit the spread of plague. Certainly so far as northwest Europe is concerned, governments were able to watch the movement of ships from infected Mediterranean ports and isolate them or refuse them entry when they arrived.[17] Whether effective or not, controls on commerce and mobility necessitated an extension of the powers of the state: more interference in civic affairs, more paperwork, more officials to collect information and enforce new regulations.

The growth of state power was even more obvious, and more far-reaching in its impact, when municipal authorities tried to deal with plague once it circumvented these protective barriers and attacked their home territory. Infected houses were identified and contact with their inmates prevented—either by removing the sick to special hospitals (pesthouses or lazarettos) or by sealing the houses with the inhabitants still inside them for a fixed period, sometimes a month, sometimes a genuine quarantine of forty days. The infected and their families had to be supported, if poor, from public funds. Finance was needed also for the fumigation or destruction of the clothes and bedding of the sick. Special officials were appointed for these tasks and special commissions—boards of health—set up to undertake the day-to-day supervision which the endeavor demanded. Not all of this was achieved at once. But in Italian towns by 1500, in the rest of western Europe by 1600, in central Europe and Russia by 1700, measures of this kind were being taken in an effort to prevent the transmission

---

[16] Biraben, *Les hommes et la peste,* 2: 86; Cipolla, *Fighting the Plague,* pp. 33–34.

[17] Biraben, *Les hommes et la peste,* 1: 231–232; Slack, *Impact of Plague,* pp. 323–326; M. W. Flinn, "Plague in Europe and the Mediterranean Countries," *Journal of European Economic History* 8 (1979): 131–48. Cf. Alexander, *Bubonic Plague in Russia,* p. 18.

of plague from person to person and household to household.[18]

This campaign had two important common features throughout Europe. First, it involved limitations on public assembly. Popular games and festivities were often banned; children were prevented from playing in the streets; in Italy there was sometimes a "general quarantine" of all who could be prevented from moving outside, especially children: they were confined to their houses. Attendance at funerals was commonly limited to a few close relatives of the deceased, and efforts were even made in some places to stop religious processions because of the danger of contagion.[19] Second, the sick and their relatives were strictly controlled. Where boards of health were most active and their regulations most sophisticated—in Italian towns—an ambitious model was recommended: the sick should be isolated in pesthouses, their contacts in other places of isolation. The empty houses should then be completely cleansed and fumigated. In cities where such expensive measures could not be undertaken, plague policy universally involved the compulsory isolation of an infected household inside its house, with doors locked, sometimes even nailed up, and food passed in through the windows.[20]

Resistance

It is perhaps unnecessary to stress that all this was ideal and

[18] For practice in Italy, see Cipolla, *Public Health*, ch. 1 *passim;* A. Carmichael, "Plague Legislation in the Italian Renaissance," *Bulletin of the History of Medicine* 57 (1983): 508–525; Cipolla, *Cristofano*, pp. 85, 168–169; Cipolla, *Fighting the Plague*, pp. 15–16; Carmichael, *Plague and the Poor*, pp. 114, 120; R. J. Palmer, "L'azione della Repubblica di Venezia nel controllo della peste," in *Venezia e la peste 1348/1797* (Venice, 1979), pp. 103–111; and for practice elsewhere: Biraben, *Les hommes et la peste,* 1: 206, 2: 103, 138–40, 169–174; Bennassar, *Recherches*, p. 47; Alexander, *Bubonic Plague in Russia*, p. 31.

[19] Cipolla, *Cristofano*, p. 99; Cipolla, *Fighting the Plague*, p. 17; Rodenwaldt, *Pest in Venedig*, pp. 56, 57, 124–125; Bennassar, *Recherches*, pp. 122–123; Carmichael, *Plague and the Poor*, p. 109; Biraben, *Les hommes et la peste*, 2: 169; Carpentier, *Orvieto*, pp. 94–95; C. M. Cipolla, *Faith, Reason and the Plague in Seventeenth-Century Tuscany* (London, 1977), pp. 47–51.

[20] Cipolla, *Fighting the Plague*, p. 68; Cipolla, *Cristofano*, pp. 29–30; Alexander, *Bubonic Plague in Russia*, p. 31; Bennassar, *Recherches*, p. 47; Slack, *Impact of Plague*, pp. 276–279.

not reality. Superhuman efforts were sometimes made: 15,000
people were reported to be in the lazarettos of Milan in the
plague of 1630; one quarter of all the households in the English
city of Salisbury were isolated at some point in the epidemic of
1604. But in a major outbreak even the richest cities could not
provide pesthouses for all the sick and their contacts; neither
could they be supported from public funds in their own homes.
In London in 1625 and again in 1665 the regulations for household isolation broke down at the height of the epidemic and the
sick were soon wandering in the streets, much to the horror of
observers like Samuel Pepys.[21] With only small police forces,
authorities could not prevent all public gatherings: "unlawful
assemblies," groups of neighbors drinking together, crowds at
funerals, were features of plague epidemics everywhere. But the
ideal existed on paper, in published regulations in town after
town in Europe; it was justified by increasing government stress
on contagion as against miasma as time went on;[22] and its publication and the attempts to enforce it in practice were sufficient
to cause controversy. For the regulations were widely resisted,
partly because all new forms of government interference were
bound to be opposed, partly, and more significantly, because
they raised issues of principle.

Some of the resistance was led by the clergy and rested on
half-concealed theological grounds. There was naturally ecclesiastical resistance to bans on religious processions or restrictions
on numbers at them: several conflicts over this issue in
seventeenth-century Italy culminated in 1630 with the pope's
excommunication of all officers of the board of health in
Florence.[23] If public religious exercises were designed to assuage

[21] Cipolla, *Cristofano*, pp. 79–80; Slack, *Impact of Plague*, pp. 278–279; R. Latham and
W. Matthews, eds., *The Diary of Samuel Pepys* (London, 1970–83), 6: 224, 233. Cf.
Alexander, *Bubonic Plague in Russia*, p. 172.

[22] Slack, *Impact of Plague*, pp. 202–203, 208; Carmichael, *Plague and the Poor*, p. 107;
Alexander, *Bubonic Plague in Russia*, p. 208.

[23] Cipolla, *Public Health*, pp. 36–37; Cipolla, *Faith, Reason and the Plague*, p. 56 and
passim. Cf. Alexander, *Bubonic Plague in Russia*, pp. 186–195 on the disorders in

God's wrath, how could they at the same time be culpable causes of contagion? On occasion, in some countries, these tensions were taken to their logical conclusion: secular precautions were seen to be incompatible with a belief in the sovereignty of divine providence. If God intended a man to die from plague, some English puritans asserted, all the precautions in the world could not save his life. Other ministers were even alleged to have said that all public-health regulations were impious, obvious interferences with God's will. It is, in fact, extremely difficult to find writers who openly expressed such views. It is easier to find examples of the ecclesiastical establishment taking an increasingly secular stance even against processions, and individual clergymen refusing to visit the infected because of the danger of contagion.[24] In general, when it came to the point, the church supported the state, and the compromise between religious and secular interpretations outlined at the beginning of this paper was maintained. But the inconsistencies within the compromise were exposed from time to time.

More serious than half-hearted appeals to divine providence, however, was the more general moral argument which some divines put forward against public-health regulations. Many of those precautions, it was correctly stated, offended against Christian charity. When people were prevented by authority from visiting their sick neighbors, attending their funerals, or comforting the bereaved, well-established social norms were being flouted; and, we might add, useful mechanisms for maintaining social cohesion in an epidemic crisis were being undermined. "Do you in this sort love your neighbour as yourself?" asked an English tract critical of prevailing measures of household-isolation: "When as at no time . . . there is greater need of fellowship, company, comfort and help, than in the time of plague." One English divine issued a similar warning: people

Moscow when efforts were made to control crowds gathering at an icon at a gate of the city.
[24] Slack, *Impact of Plague*, pp. 228–236, 286; P. Burke, *The Historical Anthropology of Early Modern Italy* (Cambridge, 1987), pp. 218, 231; Bennassar, *Recherches*, p. 31.

should not be encouraged by government to neglect "the duties of humanity" in time of plague: "For if we break these bonds I see not how human societies may continue."[25]

This indictment was especially threatening to public authority when it seemed to justify popular resistance. It is scarcely surprising that the people who suffered most from plague opposed the efforts of authority to impose control. They broke out of pesthouses and their isolated homes. They abused constables and watchmen and rubbed out the crosses which marked the doors of infected houses. All the efforts of the English government could not prevent the "meaner sort" of people in London "flocking" to funerals.[26] Not all of this resistance was altruistically motivated, of course. People broke into infected houses to loot them, as well as to visit the sick. The people who were against regulations when their own house was infected were often the first to notify the presence of infection in the house of an enemy. Epidemics were marvelous opportunities for paying off old scores. Yet there are enough references to the moral perceptions of the poor to suggest that sometimes at least there was a popular appreciation, however dim and inarticulate, that authority's reactions to epidemics of plague contradicted traditional codes of charity. The poor of London in 1637 were reported to "hold it a matter of conscience to visit their neighbours in any sickness, yea, though they know it to be the infection."[27]

The Social Dichotomy

Such arguments could make little headway, however,

[25] Slack, *Impact of Plague*, pp. 226, 309.

[26] *Ibid.*, pp. 295, 302; Biraben, *Les hommes et la peste*, 2: 117, 118; Cipolla, *Fighting the Plague*, p. 76; Cipolla, *Faith, Reason and the Plague*, pp. 30, 54; Calvi, "Metaphor for Social Exchange," pp. 151–154; J. Chartier, *La peste à Bruxelles de 1667 à 1669* (Brussels, 1969), pp. 84–88.

[27] Slack, *Impact of Plague*, p. 232.

because they were faced on the other side by a moral standpoint quite as tenacious and equally mixed with self-interest and social prejudice. The paradox is that popular resistance to regulation simply confirmed the governors in their association of plague with disorder, and particularly popular disorder, and strengthened their determination to cleanse society of all the evils which threatened public health. There is no doubt that plague regulations were designed as more than instrumental measures against contagion. They were methods of social control. In Florence they were developed at the same time as a campaign against prostitutes and beggars, other sources of pollution in the civic body. In Venice they were formulated as part of a reaction against all the diseases of the poor which seemed to threaten civic health. In England they moved hand in hand with the Poor Law and exhibited the same concerns: anyone wandering out of an infected house could be whipped as a vagrant; if he had a plague sore on him, he could be hanged as a felon. The plague-infected poor were to be incarcerated, supported, and if necessary punished in the interest both of public health and of public order, broadly defined.[28]

This interaction between fear of the poor and fear of plague was a two-way process. The threat from the poor in early modern towns seemed all the greater because they were perceived to be sources of infectious disease, not just plague, but also typhus, the "sweating sickness," and above all syphilis, that virulent "new disease" of the late Renaissance. The danger of contagion was employed to justify the new social policies of sixteenth-century municipalities. At the same time, however, the isolation procedures taken against plague would not have been so savage if the poor had not presented a conspicuous target which was subject to attack for other reasons. It is

[28] Carmichael, *Plague and the Poor*, ch. 5; B. Pullan, *Rich and Poor in Renaissance Venice* (Oxford, 1971), pp. 219–238; Slack, *Impact of Plague*, pp. 211, 303–309. Cf. Rodenwaldt, *Pest in Venedig*, pp. 55–57.

significant that plague regulations were most clearly and
strictly formulated when the socially discriminatory incidence
of the disease became conspicuous. It was not obvious in the
Black Death itself, since mortality was then so high that its
distribution seemed relatively uniform. But it was obvious by
the sixteenth century when towns were larger, the virulence of
plague less severe, and its concentration in slums and suburbs
ever more pronounced; and when long experience seemed to
have shown that the disease was often spread by beggars and
vagrants.[29] By then the social prejudices behind plague
regulations were being clearly articulated. In England the
disease was associated with the "sins of the suburbs" and of the
London poor, and respectable people prodded urban governments into taking action against them: in Norwich in 1603, for
example, the "better sort of people" were "much grieved and
offended that the under sort" would not be "restrained by the
magistrates."[30] If one is looking for social tensions in
plague-time, their most striking manifestation was not, as has
sometimes been suggested,[31] the hatred of the poor for the rich
who largely escaped infection; rather it was the contempt of
the respectable for the masses who presented a threat to their
health, their social position, and their peace of mind.

It might seem therefore that the European battle against
plague presents us with a neat social dichotomy: on the one
hand, civic rulers and patrician elites employing and enhancing state authority in order to control the threat from below;
on the other, the poor, subject to infection, striving to resist
regimentation and doing so, at least in part, in the cause of
social cohesion and the traditional moral norms which
supported it. There is certainly much in the historical evidence
which would sustain such an interpretation. But it is, in the

[29] Slack, *Impact of Plague*, pp. 192–195; Bennassar, *Recherches*, pp. 46, 53–54; Cipolla, *Fighting the Plague*, p. 53; Rodenwaldt, *Pest in Venedig*, p. 185.
[30] Slack, *Impact of Plague*, pp. 304, 306.
[31] Cf. R. Baehrel, "La haine de classe en temps d'épidemie," *Annales E.S.C.*, 7 (1952): 351–360.

final analysis, *too* neat. Social prejudice and vested interests cannot explain everything, or rather they can explain away too much. Historical circumstance is never as simple as that. If it were, it would be easy to know which side we should be on in the conflicts which arose during epidemics. In fact, of course, the threats to public health were real, and they demanded responses, even if those responses were bound to be fashioned in part by extraneous social and moral presuppositions.

Right or Wrong?

Furthermore, the measures taken against plague had, as we have seen, an empirical rationale. Their efficacy was never certain. They were far from infallible, given the limitations of contemporary medical knowledge. Some of them could even be attacked as counterproductive. It was strongly argued, for example, that shutting up the victims of plague with their families in infected houses increased rather than reduced contagion.[32] There is much to be said for that. It was and is equally plausible to argue, however, that some sacrifices had to be made for the common good. The quarantining of ships was plainly often effective. *Cordons sanitaires* around whole cities could equally succeed in protecting other towns, despite the costs it involved for those who were shut in.[33] Even the most criticized part of the program—household isolation—might on occasion serve to confine the disease to a single house or street and protect a whole town.[34] The policy was not infallible. It

[32] Slack, *Impact of Plague,* pp. 215–216, 251; Cipolla, *Public Health,* p. 61. Cf. Rodenwaldt, *Pest in Venedig,* pp. 199–200. The disputes about plague policy in Venice in 1575–76—in which two Paduan doctors argued against household sequestration and in favor of moving the poor out of the city altogether—show that while social prejudices may stimulate bureaucratic and regulatory action, they do not determine precisely what sort of action it should be: *ibid.,* pp. 180–203; Pullan, *Rich and Poor in Venice,* pp. 315–322.
[33] See the references in note 15 above.
[34] Slack, *Impact of Plague,* pp. 315, 317–319.

was open to question and dispute, and that is one of the historically interesting features of it. But it could reasonably be defended because it was likely to work.

Even with the benefit of hindsight, therefore, the plague policies pursued by early modern governments cannot be judged wholly right or wholly wrong. It is certainly possible in retrospect to try to discriminate between their various elements. We may seek to apply a cost-benefit analysis, and conclude that the social and economic expense of one procedure—household quarantine—was far greater than any likely benefit accruing from it.[35] Although such an exercise is of dubious validity, given the difficulties of investigating what would have happened if this procedure had not been employed at all, it is arguable counterfactually that mortality levels in infected towns would have been much the same without pesthouses and household isolation. But to ask contemporaries to abandon these devices is surely to ask the impossible. Given the relative success of controls on the long-distance movement of plague—on which most historians are agreed—one can scarcely criticize civic governments for locally employing isolation policies which were based on precisely the same principles.

Where there is perhaps room for retrospective judgment is in our assessment of the ways in which the policies were implemented rather than their essential strategy. If the spread of plague was to be halted, plague victims and their contacts had to be identified and access to them controlled. But how rigid should their isolation be? It is noteworthy that the English practice of total household incarceration was more ruthless than parallel procedures in the Netherlands. There the inmates of infected households were allowed visits from clergymen or specially appointed "comforters," and they were

---

[35] For an attempt at a cost-benefit analysis, see Cipolla, *Public Health*, pp. 57–66, and for some qualifications to it, Cipolla, *Faith, Reason and the Plague*, pp. 79–80.

incarcerated only during the day, being allowed out at night.[36] More flexibility of this kind could surely have been allowed than the English made room for. We might notice also the evident double standards applied in Italian towns, where only the poor were forcibly removed to crowded, anonymous plague hospitals; the rich were permitted to stay with their servants and domestic comforts at home.[37] Yet even here kindness might be cruelty in disguise. It has been reasonably argued that movement from home and therefore away from domestic rats, and the total destruction of clothing and bedding and therefore of fleas, which the practice of the best Italian lazarettos provided, were the safest precautions against the further transmission of plague.[38]

In short, no matter how much fine-tuning there might have been, hard choices had to be made. That is perhaps the greatest, if also the most obvious, lesson in the history of European responses to plague. The circumstances of epidemic disease were tragic and so were some of the consequences of the battle which was waged against. But they could not be avoided. The dilemmas were perhaps best expressed in England in the scare of 1720–22 when the disease threatened London from Marseilles. If plague arrived, the government planned to move the infected by force to pesthouses and to station troops around London and shoot anyone who escaped, in order to protect the rest of the country. There was a vast public outcry. Such measures were unnecessary, it was argued, since plague was plainly the product of local miasmas, not of

---

[36] Slack, *Impact of Plague*, pp. 210–211, 272–273; M. A. Van Andel, "Plague Regulations in the Netherlands," *Janus* 21 (1916): 412, 414.

[37] Cipolla, *Fighting the Plague*, p. 76; Biraben, *Les hommes et la peste*, 2: 169.

[38] R. J. Palmer, "The Control of Plague in Venice and Northern Italy," unpublished Ph.D. thesis, University of Kent, 1978, pp. xi, 141–143, 147, 180–182, 316–317. It is relevant to note that a modern authority on plague advocates much the same procedures in the absence of a direct attack on rats and fleas (which was not possible in the early modern period), although he also advises against the use of "forceful means" in order to obtain "the goodwill and co-operation of the people": R. Pollitzer, *Plague* (Geneva, 1954), pp. 597–598.

international contagion. They were damaging to the commerce of a trading nation. Above all, they were foreign expedients borrowed from an absolute government in France; they were totally unsuited to the "free constitution" of Britain. The plans had to be withdrawn, but not before the government's apologist, Edmund Gibson, bishop of London, had put their point forcefully: "Where the disease is desperate, the remedy must be so too," he wrote, and there was no sense in dwelling "upon rights and liberties, and the ease and convenience" of mankind, when there was "plague hanging over our heads."[39]

It was during the same crisis that Daniel Defoe, in his *Journal of the Plague Year*, reflected on the great London epidemic of 1665, on the cruel measures which had then been taken to control infection and on the popular opposition which they had aroused. He sympathized with both sides, as the historian must do, and refused to condemn either. "There was no remedy," he perceptively concluded: "self-preservation obliged the people to those severities they would not otherwise have been concerned in."[40]

Postscript

Some reflections on this essentially historical discussion of plague, in the light of other contributions to the conference, are perhaps appropriate. The most obvious difference between the societies attacked by bubonic plague in the past and the Western countries threatened by AIDS today is the difference between popular and public ignorance of the medical facts in the past and the present awareness of at least some of the features of newly discovered viruses and how they operate. Combined with modern facilities for public education and discussion in democratic societies, this knowledge holds

[39] Slack, *Impact of Plague,* p. 333.
[40] *Ibid.,* p. 337.

out the hope that responses to the threat will be more rational and more carefully planned, less haphazard and "hit or miss" than in the past. At the same time, however, the historical experience abundantly shows that reactions to threats to public health are never purely "scientific," carefully judged instrumental responses to precisely identified dangers; and they always involve restrictions on civil liberties of a more or less severe kind.

In this connection, perhaps the most important point made at the conference was that any such measures which are taken—involving, for example, the compulsory screening of certain groups in the population—must have a clearly identified useful purpose. Otherwise the opportunities for the expression of what is merely social and moral prejudice are legion. It is not for the historian to say what those measures should be. He can only suggest that the area in which prejudice and stigma are in danger of operating (or seeming to operate) should be kept as small as possible, and warn of the hard choices that have to be made and the fine-tuning that will be necessary in the application of public policies. Public debate and discussion of the kind encouraged by the contributors to "In Time of Plague" can only help that process.

IV. Moral Dilemmas— An Introduction

BY GEORGE KATEB

W E should be struck by the title of our panel, "Moral Dilemmas." At first sight it should seem odd that discussion of a particular disease lends itself to worry about moral dilemmas. After all, we usually expect that the only issue about a disease is medical: how to treat it. But as we know all too keenly, AIDS is no ordinary disease; it is not even an ordinary fatal disease. It is, rather, a disease that is contracted because of two kinds of intense pleasure: sex and drugs. This fact, by itself, would guarantee that society would take either a puritanical or a prurient interest in the disease and thus infect discussion of it with all sorts of nonmedical considerations. Whenever pleasures figure, one can also be sure that religious ideologists will take their pleasure in denouncing pleasure, and find an even greater pleasure in the fact that pleasures of a certain sort can lead to premature death. The height of religious inanity was reached by a Catholic spokesman, who said (as quoted by Robert Suro in *The New York Times*), that the church could not condone the public provision of condoms because the greatest physical harm is less important than the smallest moral harm. (This inanity, by the way, has its sources in the past, and can count Cardinal Newman as one of its authorities.) Not all the religions reach this height, but many climb quite far. The subject of AIDS, if it does nothing else, exposes the intimate connection between religion and sex (to leave aside drugs). There is something almost uncanny in the devious ways by which religion despises sex, guards it, inflames it, contorts it, sullies it, and sanctifies it. In some moods one may think that sex is all that religion is about.

The matter is yet more complicated. Because of a quirk of fortune, AIDS, in the West, turns out to have struck two groups that society dislikes and despises, male homosexuals and heroin addicts. The moral dilemmas arise because those who suffer from the disease see that even when some people in society want to understand the disease in order to help them, others, in their religious or nonreligious puritanical or prurient hostility, want to use the procedures needed to study AIDS and help those sick from it as devices of humiliation and punishment. The sick and those who may one day become sick are driven to cooperate with those who want to help them, and driven also to resist them. The sick are in a dilemma and so are those who want to help them.

Our three papers sensitively explore the main dilemma as well as other aspects of this torn situation. I would just like to point out moments in the three papers that may repay further thinking.

David Richards provides an eloquent defense of the constitutional right of homosexuals to express their sexual nature without fear of legal or social punishment. The basis of his position is the idea of human dignity, the basis of all rights, including privacy. In the course of establishing his argument, he may, however, give too large a role to "authentic feelings of affection, attachment, and mutual love." Richards's model relationship is the faithful loving couple, whether heterosexual or homosexual. His standards may be too strict. Eros is not worshiped only by faithful and loving couples. There are desires that cannot be slaked monogamously; indeed, that cannot be slaked at all, because their object is symbolic or phantasmal. Yet they are human desires, intrinsic to countless personalities, and deserve constitutional protection just as much as monogamously satisfiable desires. Not all personal integrity is monogamous. The human dignity of some people is quite compatible with, say, casual sex, or so-called "promiscuity."

Despite the overall decent good sense of Anthony Quinton's

paper, it has one chilling moment, and one hasty generalization. The chill is at the beginning, when he says that "I, like most of my reflective compatriots except for Locke, do not really believe in rights in the abstract . . . but only in legal rights and, in a more qualified fashion, in the customary rights of the members of particular historic communities." This position is in radical opposition to Richards's. Like Richards, I think that without a practice of constitutional (not merely legal or customary) rights, rooted in a vital though changeable conception of human dignity, all sorts of individuals and groups would become easier targets of harassment and persecution. Such at least is the nature of social life in America. Furthermore, Quinton's tendency is to trust political authorities a bit too much. Absolute rights, he thinks, will only get in their way. Quinton may not give enough weight to the fact that political authorities can be ruthless, which means that they move most easily in the path of least resistance (when they are not busy searching for resistance in order to overcome it). The practice of constitutional rights is a great, if leaky, barrier to oppression.

Quinton is hasty when he suggests, simply, that AIDS is contracted by voluntary action. Many homosexuals who have died from it, or now suffer from it, did not contract the disease voluntarily—that is, freely and knowingly. Many got sick before the disease was detected and identified. On the other hand, it is not common to speak of addictive behavior as voluntary.

I hope that Richard Poirier is not saying what it seems he is at one point. Is he suggesting that it would be deplorable for homosexuals and addicts if there were no "heterosexual risk factor"? I doubt that research funds would dry up if it turned out that heterosexuals were not in danger of experiencing an AIDS epidemic. The medical effort is launched worldwide.

A more general word may be in order. AIDS strikes, or is likely to strike, only a small number of people in comparison to other diseases. I do not mean to be callous when I say that the interest in it seems disproportionate from a quantitative perspective. The disproportion is a sign that the interest is charged with passions, passions of several kinds. First, there is in the background the psychological pain of the two groups most afflicted by AIDS in the West. They already suffer from society's oppressive attitudes toward them. Some of them may even suffer from self-oppression, self-reproach, a wish to be different from what they are. To these kinds of suffering is now added a terrible disease, which, even as it kills miserably, intensifies the psychological pain already present. This complex combination of pains may introduce into the situation a second sort of passion, which is pity felt by those who do not share society's oppressive outlook. Of special importance is the pity of rationalist, enlightened doctors, scientists, and lay people. When they see disease, they see only disease, see only its suffering. But when they observe that others in society are hostile to those who suffer, their vocational interest in healing may quicken; they may therefore work with an exceptional commitment. Think, for example, of Mathilde Krim. The third sort of passion in play is that of those who dislike and despise homosexuals and addicts. They welcome AIDS because it invigorates their hostility. They feel licensed, once again, to persecute and punish. As Poirier shows, they feel vindicated in their frequently murderous rejection of homosexuals and addicts. They try to spread in subtle or blatant ways two attitudes. First, let the disease rage as punishment for people who deserve what they get: death for unnatural acts and antisocial behavior. Second, if the disease is to be managed, make its management as punitive as possible; register the diseased, keep them under surveillance, inform on them, quarantine them, and generally make them feel as criminally pariah as possible.

The fact of AIDS is therefore an especially charged one. It has caused a disproportionate and intense response. Our three papers show how charged the subject is.

My own sense is that we find ourselves in a race between

enlightenment and the fundamentalist will to punish. So far, the forces of enlightenment have mostly prevailed. The public temper has been, except in notorious episodes, moderate and restrained. But if the disease spreads considerably, and still no vaccine or cure exists, then who knows? The forces of punishment could find a greater readiness in people to enact the dreams of punishment, with such phrases as "necessity" and "the public good" nicely covering punitive policies. The appeal to moral ignorance could be heeded in the void created by the helplessness of science. Such policies may do little to confine spread of the disease, or they may even spread it further, as Richards suggests. But people will have the feeling that something is being done. The will to punish and the will to save will be confusedly but inextricably joined. The bigotry of the past would once again pass as wisdom.

The despair of AIDS is a boundless subject. Think how suffering and social oppression may combine in the sufferer to produce a wish to be released that is stronger than the wish to be cured. The wish to be released may lie close to the wish to be punished. Death's termination is anticipated as erasure. The theory of rational suicide is reborn. One is haunted by what Foucault said in an interview with Robert Bono on the subject of social welfare in 1983, the year before his death:

> Foucault: . . . The idea of bringing individuals and decision centers closer together should imply, at least as a consequence, the recognized right of each individual to kill himself when he wants to under decent conditions. . . . If I won a few billion in the lottery, I would create an institute where people who would like to die would come spend a weekend, a week or a month in pleasure, under drugs perhaps, in order to disappear afterwards, as if erased.
> Bon: A right to suicide?
> Foucault: Yes.[1]

---

[1] *History of the Present* (Berkeley), no. 2 (Spring 1986): 14.

AIDS and Traditions of Homophobia

AIDS has been called a plague. But recently there have been doubts expressed that it is or will become one. Good news, if true. Meanwhile, it is of extraordinary cultural interest that these doubts are being translated into very bad—and very familiar—news about male homosexuals, still the primary victims of AIDS in this country. Theories that the AIDS epidemic will not extensively move into the heterosexual population and the fact that its rate of increase is declining among gays—both of these factors seem only to exacerbate the vituperations directed against homosexuals and, specifically, against what is assumed to be their preferred sexual practice: anal intercourse. It appears that the virus—unless it mutates— cannot be acquired by casual contact; it is contended that it cannot be easily transmitted by vaginal or oral penetration. But all this means for some is that the manner in which the virus nonetheless *can* most easily be transmitted sexually— by penetration of the anus to the point of orgasm—gives added offense to those very commentators who, it has always been assumed, are altogether unlikely to be infected in this fashion.

It is becoming clear that the stigmatization of the most likely victims of AIDS results from the fear not of physical but of moral contagion, and that the stigmatization validates itself increasingly not on medical grounds but by appeal to the most ancient of Christian abhorrences. I refer to the abhorrence of the church fathers—I doubt if this was ever shared by many of their flocks—for those forms of contraception which not only abjure abstinence but allow a promiscuous commitment to sex as a form of pleasure and not merely, or even principally, as a means of procreation. The discourse against AIDS has become increasingly a moralistic condemnation of homosexuality, empowered by the doctrinal and biblical interpretations of sex and nature that are ancient in origin and, in the Catholic and fundamentalist churches, still extremely articulate. Basically, it defines sins against nature as *any* sexual act that does not afford the maximum likelihood of procreation. It prohibits oral as well as anal intercourse between people of the same and also between people of different sex. It prohibits the position *mulier super virum,* because the woman if on top of the man was thought less likely fully to receive and retain his seed (imagine going to confession in those days?); it prohibits sex for pleasure, which means promiscuity within a marriage as well as outside it. Thus St. Thomas writes: "Whoever, therefore, uses copulation for the delight which is in it, not referring the intention to the end intended by nature, acts against nature." There must be no "disorder in the emission of seed," he says, without even having to consider emissions so wasteful as the homosexual ones.

In their designation of what is sexually unnatural, such mythologies seem grotesque and irrelevant to actual human behavior, but no more so now than they have ever been, except for the fact that the people designated as unnatural, sinful, and criminal are also dying in exceptionally horrible ways. But if AIDS increases their suffering beyond endurance it also increases the need to challenge the kind of nonsense about sex which has blighted the lives of so many millions of people over so many centuries and, quite unnecessarily, regardless of sexual preference. To expose and condemn the sexual mythologies currently at work in the discourse on AIDS ought to be undertaken in the hope that we can hand on a less cruel world than we have inherited.

Homosexuality as Disease

We are all *culture* carriers, as Barbara Rosenkrantz remarks in her chapter of this book. While thus characterizing the AIDS crisis, I am of course also aware of exceptions, of many decent responses throughout American society. Audiences, and not predominantly gay ones, have applauded dramatizations such as *The Normal Heart* or *A Quiet End* or the television dramatization *An Early Frost,* all of which vividly and sympathetically represent the plight of people with AIDS. Many in the churches (including some in the Roman Catholic hierarchy), people in the theater and the arts, in medicine, in neighborhoods where infected children have been allowed in the schools without fuss or self-congratulation—all these have acted more generously even than might have been expected. Meanwhile, gays have become a functioning community, with organizations like the Gay Men's Health Crisis that have set up services and support structures that are models for other groups who will face similar catastrophes in the future.

But the cultural odds against such efforts are formidable, sometimes overwhelming, and the odds must be addressed without illusion. The odds cannot be overcome merely by more goodwill, more contributions, or more work. In talking about AIDS and the virus which is alleged to be its primary agent, HIV (human immunodeficiency virus), I contend that the designation of the virus as the primary cause of the disease— though there are reasons to wonder if it is—has created an opportunity for a most primitive designation of homosexuality as the criminal mode of its transmission. For many powerful groups and individuals—including the U. S. Senate, members of the President's Commission on AIDS, the Vatican, the archdiocese of New York, Secretary of Education Bennett, elements of the medical profession, and some influential journals and journalists—for all these, AIDS offers an opportunity to propagate the belief (which anciently predates and is being perpetuated by the AIDS crisis) that homosexuality is itself a disease and a threat to human survival. Sometimes quite evasively, sometimes with alarming directness, these people are saying that the need to eradicate homosexuality, even as homosexuals lie dying, takes precedence over the need to eradicate the disease. To recall Susan Sontag's ever-valuable *Illness as Metaphor* and Allan Brandt's variations on her argument in his paper this morning, AIDS has become the metaphor for the *sin* of homosexuality and, more generally I think, the *sin* of sexual pleasure. Discussions of the disease—the kind of knowledge structure that is being made up with it and around it—is identical to that knowledge structure of paranoia which, for two thousand years and more, has sought to rationalize the prohibition of sexual pleasure, heterosexual as well as homosexual, when these are contrary to a human invention called "nature."

The insidious effort I am describing is helped by the fact that the etiology of the disease, its causes and the mechanisms of its transmission, remain mysterious. No one knows the originating source of the virus which is believed to cause the disease, and theories that AIDS is an advanced form of syphilis or that syphilis is a crucial cofactor, have been advanced by, among others, Dr. Peter H. Duesberg of the University of California at Berkeley, an expert on retroviruses, and by Dr. Stephen Caiazza, a New York City physician whose research, along with that of some German scientists, is discussed in an article by Katie Leishman in the January issue of *Atlantic Monthly*. The argument, briefly, is that without a cofactor, HIV would be a nonpathogenic virus. Such investigations run counter to the huge industrial and research investment in vaccines and treatments directed only at HIV, as if it were the sole cause of AIDS. The conviction the HIV is the lone culprit, working through circuits of homosexual commerce, has nonetheless allowed William F. Buckley to propose in his nationally syndicated column that all people with AIDS, as well as all asymptomatic persons infected with the human immuno-deficiency virus, should be identified and inscribed with a tattoo on forehead, genitals, and anal areas. Of course such a vicious precautionary practice would only be as efficient as the tests on which it depends, and even Buckley ought to know that no test for AIDS presently exists. Quite aside from the question of whether or not HIV is the cause of the disease or simply a cofactor, the tests now given, called ELISA and Western Blot, detect only the antibodies. These tests, which Anthony Quinton seems erroneously to think would be a dependable preliminary to quarantine, were in fact designed to screen the nation's supply of blood and plasma. They are not diagnostic. They do not identify individuals with AIDS, nor do they prove that anyone who tests positive will get AIDS in the future. According to Mark Rothstein, only 25–50 percent of seriopositive persons will develop AIDS in five to ten years. At most the test helps support a diagnosis of AIDS by its symptoms, by the presence of various opportunistic infections like pneumocystis pneumonia, Kaposi's sarcoma, or tuberculosis. Neither does it identify people with ARC (AIDS related complex) in the absence of clinical evidences like fever, diarrhea, and weight loss. It doesn't predict ARC, and only a quarter of the seriopositive persons who do not develop AIDS are predicted to develop ARC. More than that, since the test detects only antibodies stimulated by HIV, it would not identify a person as positive in the period between exposure and the development of antibodies, a process that might take anywhere from six or eight weeks to a year or more.

Even if HIV is the cause of AIDS, there is still no reliable way to infer the *active* presence of the virus from the evidence of the antibodies to it, or to infer from those antibodies that a person will eventually get AIDS or ARC. The virus is not the disease. Nonetheless, it seems clear for the present, in this country at least, that the disease has firmly established itself among certain groups, specifically homosexual men, intravenous drug users, and their sexual partners, male or female. Because these groups are already marginalized, despised, and to some extent criminalized in American society, the very mystery and uncertainty surrounding the virus has made it quite easy to add culpability, criminality, and ostracism to the devastations of the disease itself. To be a victim of AIDS is to carry a stigma, more insupportable than the "A" worn by Hester Prynne. "A" for AIDS will never be read as also meaning Able or Angel, as was Hester's "A" by a few admirers. Instead, its secondary meaning is apt to be Anus, the reproductive location of the virus, the always forbidden seat of corruption and satanic inversion. The anus figures as the bodily equivalent of the dark center of the earth, the place of insubordination and decreation. It has for centuries been imagined in this way, as in that moment in the *Inferno* when Vergil, carrying Dante on his back, makes a U-turn around the buttocks of Satan, whose lower portions are forever encased in ice. This begins the ascent which will eventually take Dante, in the *Paradiso,* to his vision of an opposing image: the rose of heaven. This rose, as Joseph Pequigney I think accurately surmises, refers to the vagina of the Virgin Mary. Love may have pitched his mansion in the place of excrement in one of Yeats's poems, but Dante and the church fathers knew that the physical proximity of the seat of waste with the source of birth required that, *conceptually,* they be placed as far away as possible from one another.

Leaving aside those who have contracted the disease from intravenous drug use—they, too, as we shall hear in a moment, are said to be victims of homosexual promiscuity—HIV is, by a wide range of commentators, so exclusively linked to anal intercourse as to suggest, in some of the phrasing, that it actually originated in and from the anus. Charged as it has always been with the particular abhorrence of the church fathers and the fundamentalists, and used, as it has always been, to mask a fear and detestation of sexual pleasure itself, anal intercourse, and the promiscuity that is mistakenly said to go with it, has moved to the center of the discourse on AIDS, especially for those who at the same time want to sustain a united front against abortion and contraception. These, too, are said to be sins against nature and forms of murder. Let me make clear that I am not denying that HIV can be transmitted by anal intercourse and that everyone should for the time being abstain from the practice. Nor need anyone be surprised by a further fact—that once a plague or a threat of plague gets linked to a sexual act of any sort, then the expectation of divine retribution follows. Even before the Christian era, plagues were almost always taken to be signs of God's displeasure for sins, often, as in the case of Oedipus, sins of a sexual kind. The plague of Thebes, you will recall, is precipitated by incest, an act also defined as unnatural. And it is immensely suggestive that the genealogy of the Theban plague in Oedipal incest parallels the genealogy of Freudian analysis. In some remarks of his on Maurice Blanchot's study of Foucault, where this conjunction is noted, Randall Havas of the Yale philosophy department recalls the remark supposedly made by Freud to Jung on the ship taking him to America: "They don't know that we bring with us the plague." Abstention from anal intercourse for medical reasons is absolutely necessary; that is not an issue any longer. Neither is the fact that human beings apparently fear, in Western culture, that sexual activity can call forth the retaliatory power of the gods. Rather, what is at issue is the rhetorical use being made of these factors. I am objecting primarily to these, and to their cultural, moral, political, and practical consequences. I am objecting to the terrible legacy which can be handed on by our response to the AIDS crisis.

The War against Homosexuality

Freud helped give a pseudoscientific credence to the ancient fear of the anus and anal intercourse, and to its importance in the creation of the new disease of homosexuality. But long before Freud, homosexuality was treated and discussed as a contagion. It is said to be latent in people, as is HIV, who do not even know they have it. And in its latency, it is always ready, supposedly, to corrupt, seduce, and betray the carrier, whenever the immune system is for any other reason most vulnerable. One of the by-now-standard journalistic inferences about the so-called Cambridge spies in British intelligence between the wars, for example, is that those recruited to serve the Comintern were already secretly members of what is archly called the Homintern. Before the act of sodomy was identified as a conduit, indeed a source, for the AIDS infection, it was already identified as a violation of the laws of God, the laws of man, and the social contract. It is against the statutes of twenty-four states and the District of Columbia. In the majority opinion upholding the state of Georgia in *Hardwick v. Bowers,* Justice Byron White said that it is merely "frivolous" to assume that the law protects the act of sodomy between consenting adults, heterosexual *or* homosexual.

Like many other terms having to do with sex, sodomy cannot be precisely defined. It can refer to fellatio or to anal intercourse, to anything involving the genitals which frustrates the impregnation of the ovum. Here St. Thomas and the Georgia courts are as one. But in the discussion of AIDS it is nearly everywhere assumed that homosexual sodomy is synonymous with anal intercourse. Given the divine and secular prohibitions of this act and the odium with which it has always been described, it is predictable that once the virus associated with AIDS got associated also with homosexual anal intercourse, then the culprit would not be the virus itself; instead, it would become homosexuality and homosexuals. Thus, measures which would frustrate the virus, like the use of condoms or, for that matter, safe sex, should not in some views even be foregrounded, since these might have the effect on less threatening occasions actually of condoning a reprehensible and forever-to-be-prohibited sexual practice. Abolish the practice rather than the virus. I see no practical difference in this respect among the positions taken by Senator Jesse Helms, Pope John Paul II, his two favorite American cardinals, Kroll and O'Connor, Patrick Buchanan, formerly on the staffs of presidents Nixon and Reagan, and more than half of the thirteen members of the President's Commission on AIDS. By a vote of 98 to 2 (the admirable Moynihan and Weicker voting against), the Senate approved a bill, introduced by Senator Helms, which denies federal funds to organizations (including the Gay Men's Health Crisis) which counsel safe sex. His argument? That it promotes what he calls "safe sodomy." The message? Abstain, or sodomize and die. So too with Cardinal O'Connor in his objections to the limited and sensible argument of other American bishops, which is that since some people are not likely to abstain from sex out of wedlock, much less homosexual sex, they should at least be told about condoms. According to his friend Cardinal Kroll, who is the American cleric closest to the pope, the AIDS epidemic is "an act of vengeance against the sin of homosexuality." He is only putting more directly what the pope himself meant when he referred to "the moral source of AIDS."

Despite this kind of thing, and worse, it is contended by some gay persons themselves, like Richard Goldstein in a recent issue of *The Village Voice*, that "AIDS has been dehomosexualized in the popular imagination." I don't know what he can mean by this unless he is making an unwarranted extrapolation from the evidence that new infections among homosexuals have dropped significantly since 1982. Safe sex seems to work; gay people have significantly policed and improved their lot. Among nearly 7,000 gay men in a continuing study of AIDS in San Francisco—it began as a study of the hepatitis B virus in 1979—the conversion from antibody negative to antibody positive in 1982 was 21 percent; in 1986, it was under 1 percent (0.8 percent); and last year, in 1987, not a single conversion occurred. The rate of increase is higher among intravenous drug users, and also among their partners, which proves, as do all statistics from Africa, and recent New York City statistics about the newborn, that the disease can be sexually transmitted by heterosexual sex as well as by anal intercourse, though not as easily. A *New York Times* editorial of December 30, 1987 mentions reports from the New York sexual disease clinics to the effect that of nearly 600 people who came in for help with sexual diseases other than AIDS, only six of those who denied being gay or drug addicted tested positive for the AIDS antibody. Since some risk factors might have been unadmitted or unknown, this means that the disease is not ready to explode, as the surgeon general warned it might, in the general population or that it deserves his comparison to the Black Death. "In other words," says the *Times,* "the AIDS epidemic may be stabilizing among gay men, it may have further spread among addicts and it has apparently not yet become self-sustaining beyond these two major risk groups and their partners." Again, however, good news of this sort—and there has since been bad news about the number of newborn babies in New York City who carry the antibodies—seems only to increase the determination of those who want to treat the epidemic more as an opportunity for war against homosexuality (and promiscuity) than against the virus. A well-orchestrated example of such determination was evident in two recent, successive issues of *Commentary* magazine, edited by that historic homophobic, Norman Podhoretz.

The first, by a journalist named Michael A. Fumento, appeared in the November 1987 issue and was titled "AIDS: Are Heterosexuals at Risk?" (his answer, two months ago, was no); the other, in the December issue, is by a psychotherapist named Marjorie Rosenberg, entitled "Inventing the Homosexual," as if a bunch of celibate priests along with other interested parties have not for centuries been inventing "the heterosexual." Fumento's well-conducted argument is meant to prove that AIDS will remain lodged within the self-infecting groups where it is currently taking its toll. That being his conviction, why must he then beat up on them even more, as with the smart-aleck suggestion that because homosexual-rights groups are aware of "the appeal exercised by the notion that AIDS is nature's or God's retribution on them they have sought to tie AIDS to heterosexual sex"? That particular achievement belongs to the World Health Organization (not known to be a homosexual-rights group), a surgeon general well known for his conservative views on abortion, the National Institutes for Health, and the researchers for the Centers for Disease Control. At the end, Fumento insists that from now on every commercial must stress that "promiscuous anal intercourse and needle sharing are the overwhelming risk factors in the transmission of AIDS." But the predictable effect of such an emphasis would be to pretend that the heterosexual risk factor does not exist, which no one even after Fumento's adroit figuring should dare to concede, and it would mean that all funding for such commercials, and for most research—only to save faggots and drug abusers?—would dry up. Recall that Senator Helms has already counted ninety-eight Senate votes against paying for anything that leads to "safe sodomy."

Fumento's essay sets the statistical and political ground for the piece by Rosenberg. Hers is an altogether less impressive performance, full of question-begging, harrumphing moralism, and the by now ritual attacks on homosexual promiscuity and anal intercourse, as if anyone, under present conditions, is ready to promote either of these. The insinuating, ghettoizing tone of the Rosenberg and Fumento arguments—particularly unbecoming in a magazine supported by people on the American Jewish Committee who know very intimately about the historical persecution of minorities—can only deflect energy and attention away from practical measures, even while it frightens already very frightened people who need every encouragement to come forward if they are to receive counseling and experimental treatment.

The scapegoating of such pieces is the more dangerous for its rhetorical claims to moral rectitude and intellectual cool. No less so, it is necessary to add, is the sprightly pretense to dispassion by which the philosopher from Oxford on this panel, Anthony Quinton, expresses his concern less for AIDS victims that for the insurance companies who might have to pay their medical and death benefits. His modest proposal is that the infection can fairly be considered the result of "voluntary actions from which [the victim] could have abstained," so that it can be argued that the victim has no more rights to insurance payments than would a suicide who only recently took out a policy. Leaving aside the various meanings of "voluntary," why not apply the same principle to anyone who gets into a fatal accident after drinking an immoderate amount of alcohol? Or to anyone who willingly exposes herself, even in the care of loved ones, to an infection known to prove fatal? The "voluntary" principle is especially grotesque in the case of AIDS because many of its victims, and probably most of them, picked up the virus even before it was known to exist; and since its incubation period can be as long as ten years, many more who carry it cannot in any sense have "volunteered" to get it. An argument so specious is not to be understood as mere speculative solicitude for Lloyds of London.

The writers in *Commentary,* and others who more indirectly share their view, all exhibit, you will notice, nothing of the fear and terror that these two writers and others who share their views exhibit, nothing of the fear and terror that provoked earlier scapegoating during the onset of plagues, as in the flagellant processions and the intensifications of the pogroms against the Jews during the Black Death in the middle of the fourteenth century. There are, to be sure, evidences here and in England of an equivalent fear and terror about AIDS. Some people in Arcadia, Florida, everyone knows, burned down the pathetically wretched home of a family whose three small hemophiliac boys had developed AIDS, and a house in London was recently torched by neighbors who knew that its two inhabitants had AIDS. But if there is a choice between the arsonists in Arcadia and the intellectualists in *Commentary* and elsewhere, it is a choice only between fire and ice. And the ice is neither very clear nor very sparkling. What, for example, is anyone expected to *do* about AIDS when told by Ms.

Rosenberg that "To the Greeks it would have been inconceivable that free men would choose to engage in such activities"? I would suggest, to paraphrase a much shrewder woman when it comes to sex, that freedom had nothing to do with it. And how are we possibly to take the anatomically startling reassurance from Mr. Fumento, never to be outdone in the glorification of free men, that "some sort of passageway is needed [for the virus] and in the case of most Americans such passageways do not exist"? Reassuring, I suppose, especially when it might be thought that we had become a nation of such passageways!

Any doubts as to the political intention behind the serial publication of these two pieces in *Commentary* was dispelled by the use made of them by Patrick Buchanan. Not that he needs help on the subject, having already written two syndicated columns in May 1983 entitled "AIDS Disease: It's Nature Striking Back." In his column for December 2, 1987, he gives repeated credit to the Fumento piece—and by then he had doubtless read the Rosenberg—in order to put the position shared by all three with brutal directness: "There is only one cause of the AIDS crisis," he writes,"—the willful refusal of homosexuals to cease indulging in the immoral, unnatural, unsanitary, unhealthy, and suicidal practice of anal intercourse, which is the primary means by which the AIDS virus is being spread through the 'gay' community, and thence into the needles of drug abusers, the transfusions of hemophiliacs, and the blood streams of unsuspecting health workers, prostitutes, lovers, wives, and children. By the way they define themselves, i.e., by anonymous and promiscuous sex, the unbridled homosexuals are killing themselves and killing others as well . . . Anal intercourse—buggery—the defining practice of the homosexual, is uniquely suited by human nature for the spreading of the AIDS virus. The only way to stop the epidemic is to stop the sodomizing." In fact, anal intercourse is not the "defining practice of homosexuals" except in the paranoid fantasies of male heterosexuals like Buchanan. The predominant practice even before AIDS was mutual masturbation and fellatio, which also accounts for the famed (or infamous) capacity of more active homosexuals for multiple scores in one evening. Obviously, under present conditions, mutual masturbation and fellatio, usually with a condom, is even more the custom. The idea that if sodomizing stopped so would the epidemic is nonsense, as if sodomy gave birth to the virus in some grotesque impregnation of the anus or that it is responsible for its transmission by needles.

Buchanan really does not want a cure for AIDS, he wants a cure for anal intercourse. Is there one? Perhaps. Since, in his attack on promiscuity and sexual practices which are against nature, he depends so implicitly on the church fathers, Buchanan ought to read more deeply in the works of one of them, Albertus Magnus. In the synthesis of theology and canon law begun by the church in the middle of the thirteenth century—a synthesis which clearly remains potently at work in the twentieth—Albertus was the first to comment extensively on what came to be called homosexual behavior. Such behavior offended "grace, reason, and nature" more so than adultery, which offended, he said, only the first two. He describes sodomizing as a contagious disease, very hard to get rid of. However—and here I will quote from James Boswell's *Christianity, Social Tolerance, and Homosexuality*—"in his treatise on animals he described an easy cure: the fur of the neck of an Arabian animal he called 'alzabo,' burned with pitch and ground to a fine powder, would cure a 'sodomite' to whose anus it was applied." Albertus was using, without knowing it, a transliteration into Latin of an Arabic word which means "hyena," a fact that might have embarrassed him, since in vulgar tradition the hyena itself was considered homosexual. This could hardly have been consistent with his claim that sodomy was an act contrary to nature.

It is not for us, however, to speak condescendingly of the past, not when we have William F. Buckley's tattoos to our credit, or the recommendation of the publisher of *The Saturday*

Evening Post, Cory Ser Vaas, who, with John Cardinal O'Connor, is one of the thirteen members of the President's Commission on AIDS. She told the *New York Native* that she hopes scientists will discover "the genetic predisposition to being homosexual so we could minimize that behavior thereby reducing AIDS." Again, the same illusion: that if you can only get rid of homosexuality you will get rid of or reduce AIDS. In this view, the cure is not medical; it is moral, in line with the always presumptuous Christian notion that facts of nature are no more than the moral facts we have invented to stand duty for nature. The effort to turn the AIDS crisis into a renewed campaign against sexual practices of a contraceptive kind, and thus into a punitive campaign against homosexuality, will only delay and frustrate any effort to control and end this nightmare disease, to isolate and disarm a virus whose mutations, if we fail to go after it now and directly, might in time, as Joshua Lederberg's paper starkly reminds us, become a threat to human reproductive survival, and which even in its present form is already producing its antibodies in one out of sixty-one newborn babies in New York City.

Plagues and
Morality

BY ANTHONY QUINTON

As soon as the idea takes hold, rightly or wrongly, that a disease can be communicated by sufferers to people who are not infected, an array of morally significant reactions is provoked in those who entertain the idea. The most straightforward response is to prevent the contact through which the disease might be communicated. The practically simplest way of eliminating contact is to segregate the infected from the rest of the community. That, of course, was the rule laid down in the book of Leviticus to contain the spread of leprosy. From the point of view of effectiveness it was not a bad scheme, given that leprosy appears to be communicated from one person to another by close and prolonged physical contact. The additional sufferings it imposed on lepers, however, at least invite the question whether there might not be some less draconian way of achieving the same result.

Isolation of sufferers already within a community is one thing; the exclusion of bearers of disease, actual or possible, from entering the community is another. That is what we first think of, I suppose, when we encounter the word *quarantine*. I start from this ancient example of response to a plague because we are trying here to view lethal epidemics in part in a historical way and also because a few years ago some public-opinion survey conducted by the *Los Angeles Times* recorded that 51 percent of the respondents were in favor of quarantining AIDS sufferers. The isolation of sufferers from a disease is obviously pointless if it can be or usually is communicated by someone who carries the agent of infection without showing any signs of the fact. That is the case with measles. It is also a very conspicuous feature of AIDS. The HIV virus can be carried for years without manifesting itself in the form of visible symptoms in its carrier.

The period of incubation is just one of the dimensions along which epidemic diseases may vary. Another is their mode of transmission: whether by infected human beings (as with smallpox and typhoid) or by mosquitoes (as with malaria and yellow fever) or by fleas dwelling on infected rats (as with plague proper). Isolation is altogether useless to contain diseases spread by nonhuman carriers. Sanitation is what is needed. Other dimensions are: their amenability to treatment, the degree of their fatality, their susceptibility to containment by inoculation.

The different modes of transmission of diseases means that there will be great differences between what it is *sensible* to do to prevent their spread, quite apart from the question of what it is morally acceptable to do. That question arises only about courses of action which come up for serious consideration, in virtue of being well judged to bring about a result acknowledged to be good, and concern the human costs of the side effects of the beneficial courses of action.

Rights of the Diseased

If there were such things as rights of the diseased in general they would have to be of a very vague and flexible nature to allow for these differences. I, like most of my reflective compatriots except for Locke, do not really believe in rights in the abstract, the rights of human beings at all times, everywhere and in all circumstances, but only in legal rights and, in a more qualified fashion, in the customary rights of the members of particular historic communities. That does not imply that I claim not to understand, or pretend not to use, the vocabulary of human rights in general. But I interpret statements about such rights as statements about what human beings generally ought to be allowed to do or be provided with, so long as there is no overwhelming reason why they should not. To invoke, for example, a human right of privacy to rule out a course of action which would serve some admittedly good purpose is not, in my view, to end the matter by the production of some kind of argumentative trump card. It is not self-evident that the protection of privacy should always outweigh other considerations. But that is not to deny that privacy is important to human beings for a number of reasons, which include, but go beyond, the fact that they have a strong desire for it. Nor is it to deny that privacy is a significant value which requires there to be substantial reasons for its invasion if it is to be invaded.

There is no need here to get entangled in the investigation of the nature of moral rights in general. What I would claim is that discussion of the moral aspects of epidemic disease cannot be rationally carried on in terms of a handful of absolute or categorical principles of right, which are taken to fix unalterable limits to acceptable courses of action. To put the point in another way, consideration of the moral aspects of disease must concern itself not just with the intrinsic character of proposed courses of action but also with the consequences of action compared with those of abstaining from action. These consequences will concern a long period of time and (since we are dealing with social policies, not single human actions) they will be complicated and various.

To arrive at a view about the long-run consequences of policies involves predictions which rest on the available stock of relevant theory. These will often be more or less tentative and insecure. The history of movements of belief and opinion in the still-short period of the AIDS crisis brings this out clearly. The state of well-founded information about the nature of the disease has changed constantly since it was first identified at the beginning of the decade. The matter has been complicated, furthermore, by a good deal of lack of candor and rhetorical exaggeration, conducted in the interests of what are conceived as persecuted minorities on the one hand and for the sake of reinforcing traditional rules of sexual behavior on the other. Thus the minimal danger to male heterosexuals who have ordinary sexual intercourse with women who have been infected by primary carriers of the virus has been denied or obscured. One end pursued by doing so is to awaken the interest, concern, and readiness to bear costs of the great majority of the population which is not in fact dangerously at risk. Another, ideologically opposite, aim is to terrify people into thinking that they are at risk if they make any departure from strict, life-long monogamy.

Let us begin by considering the main methods of controlling epidemic diseases to see what moral problems arise. The least troublesome is sanitation, the only way to control malaria and yellow fever, the best way to control typhoid. Effective sanitary policies involve interfering with people's habitual practices of hygiene and refuse disposal and so could, by a very dim-witted or obstinate libertarian, be regarded as infringements of freedom. Property owners will be compelled to get rid of swamps or, at least, to allow them to be got rid of.

Another great historic controller of disease has been inoculation or immunization. It has largely eliminated small-pox and polio and has made effective inroads into diphtheria, influenza, and measles. There is a modest negative aspect to shots. They are inevitably a nuisance to turn up for. They may be anything from very faintly to acutely painful. They may produce unpleasant reactions. In rare cases they may lead to contracting the disease they were intended to protect one from. Fifty years ago in Britain up to half the population was not vaccinated against smallpox because of what was described as "conscientious objection." I think that a way of avoiding vaccination was provided to accommodate people who had a deep-seated religious objection to the process. The large numbers availing themselves of the escape clause must have been almost entirely composed of people who could not be bothered (I believe it was provided free of charge).

Immunization, then, is no more than a nuisance and only very faintly dangerous. It falls equally on everyone. Other disease conditions invite much greater interference and a measure of what may seem to be objectionable selectivity. One example is venereal disease, which has often been met with the legally compulsory inspection of prostitutes. In Britain in the 1860s a series of contagious diseases acts were passed which required the registration, licensing, and medical examination of prostitutes in eighteen towns where there were large numbers of soldiers and sailors. The object was to increase the efficiency of the armed forces. When the idea of applying the procedure to the whole country was proposed, an agitation against the laws began which succeeded in getting them suspended in 1883 and repealed in 1886.

John Stuart Mill and other campaigners for repeal argued principally that the law discriminated unfairly against women, by subjecting them to interferences and indignities to which the men who had recourse to them were not submitted. Servicemen had previously been inspected and are, I imagine, inspected at intervals now. They certainly were during the war, as I can attest from repeated personal experience, even when most of those involved were conscripts, and I know of no outcry or even criticism of the procedure.

The most extreme public interference with ordinary claims of right is the ancient practice of isolation or quarantine. This has persisted for people seeking to enter a country from outside and was a major—indeed, often practically unbearable—inconvenience until brought within reasonable bounds by international agreements in the mid-nineteenth century. It is at least sensible or relevant to apply it to infected people if they are the main carriers of the disease or to those who have been in contact with its prime sources, if they are, or will, after the incubation period, be the main carriers.

A notorious instance of this was the case of Mary Mallon, or

"Typhoid Mary," incarcerated in North Brother Island, off the Bronx, for most of the thirty-year period before her death in 1938. She was a carrier of the disease, but herself immune to it. Her determination to work as a cook made her a public danger, together with her resolute efforts to avoid sequestration. It may be suspected that her personal hygiene left something to be desired as well, since a small but significant proportion of those who contracted the disease remain long-term carriers of it after recovery, but do not do the damage she did. There can hardly be a more conspicuous instance of the sacrifice of an individual to the welfare of the community as regards epidemic disease than Typhoid Mary.

Social Policy

I want to turn now to the bearing of these general considerations on the AIDS epidemic. AIDS has some distinctive peculiarities which must be taken into account.

The first is that it is in the very great majority of cases transmitted by bodily contact, in particular by bodily contact of a rather rough or invasive kind, in which the blood, semen, and, just possibly, the saliva of an infected person gets through the skin, by way of some lesion, of someone else. Otherwise it can be communicated by infected blood introduced by transfusion or by inheritance from an infected mother.

The second is that it has a very long incubation period. One fairly tentative survey I know of estimates the average as three years. But a larger figure was mentioned at a previous session. That, of course, means that there are likely to be many people who are infected without being aware of the fact.

The third is that the disease is incurable and—which is not quite the same thing—once contracted, always leads within a reasonably short period to death.

Finally, there is no real therapeutic treatment for it, only measures for the alleviation of symptoms, and there seems to be no immediate possibility of finding some kind of vaccine to immunize people against it.

The first distinguishing mark implies that sanitary measures are not relevant in the way they are to insect-borne diseases caused by dirty food and water. Furthermore, AIDS is not, as are droplet infections, easy to pick up through everyday proximity to infected people. Like venereal disease, there has, in most cases, to be literal bodily contact, and, unlike venereal disease, the contact has to be of a very forceful or vehement nature.

The second feature implies that for any sort of isolation or quarantining to be effective it would have to be applied not just to the large enough group of those actually suffering from AIDS or AIDS-related diseases but to the very much larger group of those with the virus in their bodies. Since most of them do not know it is there, there would have to be a screening of a very large part of the total population— everyone up to the age of the end of sexual activity.

I suppose most public concern about the control of AIDS at the moment is focused on allowing sufferers to attend schools, to continue in work which involves comparatively close contact with others, and to be present as employees or as clients at restaurants and other places of public resort. The concern is understandable; people naturally assimilate a new medical threat to familiar ones. But it is doubly misplaced. In the first place, to exclude only those suffering from AIDS and AIDS-related diseases from schools and the like would be to leave out all the other carriers of the virus, the very much larger number who have not yet fallen ill and, indeed, may not do so. Second, and more conclusively, ordinary social proximity, even if it involves mild bodily contact, has nothing to do with the spread of the virus.

Screening or testing is another matter. To screen immigrants is not, to the best of my knowledge, a proposal that has been widely discussed. But it would be in line with policies that have been adopted by many states without drawing obloquy on themselves. It is continuous with, though stronger than, the formerly rather common requirement that foreigners coming into a country, for a visit as well as permanently, should bring with them a recent certificate of vaccination.

Given that three-quarters at present of those who contract AIDS are male homosexuals, there is something to be said for screening those who are in institutions in which homosexual rape, or something amounting to it, is prevalent. All prisoners should be screened, as should all servicemen (as they are in the United States, even if not for this reason). It also seems reasonable to suppose that intravenous drug use of the social and lethally dangerous kind which involves the sharing of needles will be more common in enclosed male communities like prisons and barracks.

What should be done with those found to be HIV positive in such establishments? If prisoners, they should be segregated; if servicemen, discharged (as they are in the United States, with an honorable medical discharge). Should they be? The two cases are different. The element of stigma is minimized by returning the virus-carrying servicemen to the general population; it is maximized by confining HIV-positive prisoners in special prisons, AIDS leprosaria. The object could be achieved less offensively by having special wings for the HIV-positive in some prisons. There remains the depressing thought of the prospects in such a place of a young prisoner whose HIV positivity was inherited or acquired from a transfusion.

The screening of blood donors, together with the heat treatment for blood, would seem capable of eliminating transfusion-borne infection in a short time and completely and not, in the developed world, at intolerable cost. In general there are two patterns of blood donation; it is motivated either by simple public-spiritedness or by the desire for payment. The public spirit that sustains the former practice should extend without difficulty to include readiness to be screened.

In the latter we have a commercial transaction whose terms need to be altered, one which donors are free to accept or refuse.

The problem of infected blood in the undeveloped world is much more serious in that a large proportion of the blood available for transfusion is infected. (Medical needles, as well as drug users' needles, are also carriers of infection.) As a moral problem there is nothing special about this. It is part of the general problem of the responsibilities of richer nations to give support to poorer ones. Since most such aid is financed by compulsorily extracted taxation, a secondary responsibility is incumbent on governments giving it to see that it is used effectively for the purposes for which it was extracted in the first place. It is seldom clear that they are in a position to discharge this responsibility and keep faith with their citizens.

A particular problem that arises about AIDS is that of the conditions under which life-insurance coverage should be given to the infected and benefits paid to their beneficiaries. It is normal and accepted practice for insurance companies to adjust their premiums according to the best estimates they can make of the life expectancy of those seeking insurance. In a system of competitive insurance provision, those firms that do not do this will go out of business. People with poor expectancies will insure with them; those with good expectancies will insure with those who fit the level of premium to expectation.

It could be argued that it is unfair to penalize naturally unfortunate people—or, more properly, their dependents— for the fact that they are likely to die sooner than most people. I have not encountered the argument, but it seems to me not without force. Nevertheless, it applies only weakly to the case in hand. Someone with a congenital disease from which he will die young does not do so as a result of voluntary actions from which he could have abstained. But that is the case with most— although, of course, by no means all—of those who suffer from AIDS. In the present state of knowledge, anal intercourse and needle-sharing, if not quite suicide, are more than half way to it: a kind of hyper-Russian roulette. Insurers often will not pay out for suicides if they occur in less than some number of years after the policy was taken out. To take out a policy with the intention of committing suicide is, in effect, fraud.

It has been judged by some to be an unjustifiable invasion of privacy for insurers to ask applicants if they are homosexual or are intravenous drug users. It is plainly not efficient. The annoyance it will generate would only enhance a predictable lack of candor about such intimate and, indeed, rather shady subjects. Screening would be more efficient and less intrusive. Another possibility would be for insurers to follow the policy I mentioned about suicide. That would take rational account of those who are infected without knowing it, without intrusion or any implication of blame. It still adds impoverished beneficiaries to early death as part of the fate of an AIDS victim. But there is no compelling reason to break this connection in this kind of case, while leaving it in place where there is no voluntary element in the incurring of the misfortune.

A complicating factor in considering the moral aspects of AIDS is that something like 90 percent of those who contract the disease are homosexuals practicing anal intercourse or drug takers. Sodomy and drug taking have long been prohibited by law, and that prohibition reflected a long-lasting moral consensus which, in the Western world, was rooted in Judeo-Christian religion. Sodomy is now legalized here and there within certain limits. Where it remains illegal no great effort is put into its suppression. AIDS is contracted, not only by voluntary action, but by voluntary action of a kind which is legally forbidden and still rather widely morally deplored, even if it is not the object of the kind of intense moral outrage it used to be.

There is surely no doubt that if AIDS were caused by some absolutely morally neutral activity like eating cod's roe or drinking goat's milk most people would feel a little differently about it. That is perhaps in part because giving up cod's roe or goat's milk seems something exceedingly easy to do. In the circumstances imagined, therefore, anyone who went on with them would be regarded as deranged. Homosexuality and drug taking are altogether deeper; a constitutional propensity, in one case, an addiction in the other. But that is not the whole story.

If a robber and the store owner he is seeking to rob wound each other nonfatally, do we not feel that—other things like the severity of their wounds being equal—the storekeeper should be the first to receive medical attention, although not the only one, of course? I suspect that members of high-risk groups take some such principle to be implicit in the general public's often unsympathetic attitude to AIDS. To the extent that it is, it needs to be brought into the open. Law tends, on the whole, to reflect prevailing morality or, at least, what prevailed a little while ago. That is one reason, although it is not the only reason, why it is morally obligatory to obey the law. (Let me hasten to add that I do not regard this obligation as absolute or indefeasible.) But morality is not of uniform texture. The wrongness of robbing a store with lethal weapons is part of the central, compulsory core of morality which is not seriously disputable. Homosexual behavior and drug taking are in a quite different position. Hostility to the former is really an expression of distaste. There is no recognized array of acknowledged bad consequences to which it is supposed to lead. As for drug taking, it is of many very different kinds, some harmful to none, some harmful only to the drug takers themselves, all harmful to anyone else only by way of secondary effects arising from social attitudes to drug taking (stealing to finance the habit and so forth).

Earlier I used the word *shady* to characterize the marginal moral status of homosexuality and drug taking, intending it to cover a considerable measure of moral disapproval in the community at large as well as the very peripheral character of that disapproval. For anyone who sees them as no more than a bit disreputable, let alone as innocent, and not as wicked, the misfortunes of their practitioners cannot reasonably sustain the implications of priority of concern that do appear appropriate in the case of the robber and the storekeeper.

Individual Behavior

The moral issues considered so far have all been concerned with social policy as opposed to individual behavior. It might be expected that problems of the second kind might arise for doctors and for those suffering from AIDS and AIDS-related diseases or who know themselves to be HIV-positive—in other words, the infected. I do not see that doctors have a special problem with confidentiality. If insurance companies, school boards, prospective employers, and so forth ask for information which can serve no actual purpose in protecting people from the disease, doctors should simply refuse, with a clear conscience, to supply the information required. It is vital for trust between doctors and AIDS victims to be preserved. Although doctors cannot cure sufferers, they can, it seems, prolong life for some with AZT, and can contribute effectively to making the grim progress of the disease significantly less terrible than it might be without them.

But doctors surely should tell victims, and all the infected indeed, that they are in that condition. Holding back an agonizing truth is perhaps permissible where a lethal disease— cancer of the liver, for example—is not communicable. The situation is altogether different where the person from whom the truth about himself is withheld may thus be prevented from giving up the behavior which spreads his complaint to lovers and friends.

For that communication of trust to do the good it is capable of, it is, of course, necessary that the infected should recognize that they ought, for the sake of others, to stop doing things which carry an appreciable risk of consigning those others to a painful death, long before a more normal date for the end of their lives. The closeness of members of the two high-risk groups to those they are likely to harm, itself a consequence of the way in which the disease is acquired, is a reason for hoping that this obligation will be widely recognized and contribute to the stemming, or even reversal, of the tide of the disease.

Human Rights, Public Health, and the Idea of Moral Plague*

BY DAVID A. J. RICHARDS

I T is a distinctive feature of Western ethics and law that the best standards of argument in both areas are cultivated by self-critical methodologies of historiography, empirical science, and ethical reflection. We insistently reflect on the history of our ethics and law, and think of such reflection as part of a larger process of cultural self-criticism through which we identify those strands of our tradition worth preserving and elaborating (for example, respect for the essential liberties of free people committed to democratic processes under the rule of law) and those strands that we now reject (for example, slavery and the subjection of women).

At the center of this self-critical enterprise is a creative tension between its affirmative and negative components, for we often best understand the point of our most enduring values when we see how they often flourished in uncritical tension with our gravest moral corruptions and political failures. We may better understand, for example, liberty of conscience as an ethical and legal value when we see how Augustine, on the one hand, offered a philosophical psychology supportive of freedom of conscience as an ultimate value and, on the other hand, defended a theory of persecution quite inconsistent with such freedom;[1] our constitutional tradition's rejection of Augustine's theory of persecution is thus understood as a self-critical rejection of a corruptive moral argument that undermined a defensible ethical and legal ideal.[2] Correspondingly, we may better grasp our own ethical and political responsibilities now if we can frame our central contemporary dilemmas by critical reflection that both constructively elaborates the central principles of ethics and law at stake and exposes our recurrent temptations to moral corruption for what they are.

There is no more fruitful topic for such inquiry than the dilemmas that surround the AIDS health crisis, including our very temptation to frame the discourse in the historical terms of the social response to plagues. I will, in the course of this essay, offer reasons to reject such terms of discourse precisely because its motivation, the idea of a moral plague, is not merely an outmoded myth but, in Susan Sontag's sense,[3] an obfuscating metaphor of illness false to fact and ideologically freighted with moral and political corruption; it is morally and politically irresponsible, so I shall argue, to give any weight to this pernicious conceptual anachronism in contemporary circumstances. There are genuine dilemmas that surround response to the AIDS health crisis, but the idea of moral plague is not one of them. Rather, the irrational political force that the idea enjoys conflicts with the principles that should govern these issues.

It is fundamental to our dilemma that our legitimate public-health concerns for control of a deadly virus center in the United States on the populations at highest risk[4] and that

---

[1] For pertinent discussion and citations, see David A. J. Richards, *Toleration and the Constitution* (New York: Oxford University Press, 1986), pp. 58–88.

[2] *Ibid.*, pp. 89–141.

[3] See Susan Sontag, *Illness as Metaphor* (New York: Vintage, 1977), p. 3.

[4] One study reports that the distribution of AIDS cases in the United States is more than 70 percent among homosexuals and 17 percent among intravenous drug users: see Institute of Medicine, National Academy of Sciences, *Mobilizing Against AIDS* (Cambridge, Mass.: Harvard University Press, 1986), p. 121.

these populations, on independent ethical and/or legal grounds, increasingly call upon our concern against abusive state authority. I focus in my discussion here on homosexuals and their rights to both privacy and antidiscrimination because the level of ethical and constitutional argument is fairly well advanced,[5] albeit yet unsuccessful at the highest judicial level.[6] But comparable arguments could fairly be developed both for IV drug users[7] and the racial and ethnic minorities[8] that constitute many of those users.[9] We need a clear understanding of human rights and to what extent homosexuals' claim to such rights are just in order to frame the corresponding issues of public health.

Human Rights and Overcriminalization

It is now common ground among Western liberal democracies that their governing political theory imposes significant constraints of human rights on the scope of state coercive

[5] See, e.g., Richards, *Toleration and the Constitution*, pp. 269–280.

[6] In *Bowers v. Hardwick*, 106 S. Ct. 2841 (1986), the Supreme Court decided, in a 5–4 opinion, that the constitutional right to privacy did not encompass consensual homosexual acts. For criticism of the decision, see David A. J. Richards, "Constitutional Legitimacy and Constitutional Privacy," *New York University Law Review* 61 (1986): 800. The narrow majority of the Supreme Court and the well reasoned and cogent dissenting opinions reflect a remarkable shift in the Court's approach to these matters from its summary affirmance of a dismissal of comparable claims in 1976; see *Doe v. Commonwealth's Attorney*, 403 F. Supp. 1199 (E. M. Va. 1975), *aff'd without opinion* 425 U. S. 901 (1976). In this essay, I support the argument of the dissenting opinions.

[7] See, in general, Harold M. Ginzburg, "Intravenous Drug Abusers and HIV Infections: A Consequence of Their Actions," *Law, Medicine and Health Care* 14 (1986): 268.

[8] See, e.g., Wayne L. Greaves, "The Black Community," in Harlon L. Dalton et al., eds., *AIDS and the Law* (New Haven: Yale University Press, 1987); Nancy Mueller, "The Epidemiology of the Human Immunodeficiency Virus Infection," *Law, Medicine and Health Care* 14 (1986): 252.

[9] Indeed, such arguments might have special force in view of the powerlessness of IV drug users in contrast to a comparatively well organized and militant gay community. On the latter, see Ronald Bayer, "AIDS and the Gay Community: Between the Specter and the Promise of Medicine," *Social Research* 52 (1985): 58.

power over the lives of persons. John Stuart Mill's *On Liberty* influentially formulated these constraints in a general doctrine that may be termed the "harm principle": subject to background duties of justice and fair contribution, the coercive power of the state can only be imposed on acts causing harms to other persons, and harms to self do not suffice.[10] American constitutional law has elaborated a related form of argument in the form of the constitutional right to privacy that imposes a heavy burden of justification comparable to Mill's harm principle on the coercive power of the state over activities protected by the right to constitutional privacy. The Supreme Court of the United States has, for example, extended such protection to the sale and use of contraceptives,[11] access to abortion services,[12] the use of pornography in the home,[13] though not to homosexual sexuality as such.[14] In my analysis here, I briefly offer an argument elaborated at greater length elsewhere[15] that both explains and defends the constitutional right to privacy in general and its proper application in particular not only to contraception use and abortion services but to consensual adult homosexuality. I begin with an examination of why the constitutional right to privacy is a natural and principled elaboration of our constitutional traditions, and then turn to why it properly applies to consensual homosexuality.

---

[10] See, in general, John Stuart Mill, *On Liberty* (New York: Appleton-Century-Crofts, 1947). Many liberals no longer agree with the stringent form of Mill's formulation of the harm principle, for example, his prohibition on all paternalistic arguments. See, e.g., H. L. A. Hart, *Law, Liberty, and Morality* (Stanford: Stanford University Press, 1963), pp. 30–34. For a plausible contemporary restatement of Mill's harm principle, with which I largely agree, see Joel Feinberg, *Harm to Others* (New York: Oxford University Press, 1984), pp. 1–27; idem, *Offense to Others* (New York: Oxford University Press, 1985), pp. ix–xiv; idem, *Harm to Self* (New York: Oxford University Press, 1986), pp. ix–xviii.

[11] *Griswold v. Connecticut*, 381 U. S. 479 (1965).

[12] *Roe v. Wade*, 410 U. S. 113 (1973).

[13] *Stanley v. Georgia*, 394 U. S. 557 (1969).

[14] *Bowers v. Hardwick*, 106 S. Ct. 2841 (1986).

[15] See Richards, *Toleration and the Constitution,* pp. 231–281.

The Constitutional Right to Privacy. The constitutional right to privacy is probably the most widely criticized recent development in constitutional interpretation. These criticisms include the claim that the right is improperly nontextual and thus noninterpretivist, that it wrongly confuses constitutionally protected privacy interests with autonomy interests not protected by the Constitution, and that it wrongly confuses valid liberal political argument (properly effectuated through normal democratic processes) with constitutional arguments of principle not the proper subject of political bargaining and compromise.[16] None of these arguments is, I believe, valid as a matter of sound constitutional history, interpretation, or political theory; indeed, they fail to take seriously the central place of toleration as an organizing principle of our constitutional traditions. Let me briefly suggest why this is so as a preface to a constructive sketch of the provenance and nature of the constitutional right to privacy in our law.

It is simply not the case that the constitutional right to privacy is a nontextual and thus noninterpretivist right, for it is abundantly clear historically that the Founders were very concerned indeed that any rights specified in a Bill of Rights would lead to the improper inference that other rights of the person—clearly immune from the scope of just state concern— were not constitutionally immune from state power. Indeed, it was precisely this argument which justified the objection of leading Founders like Hamilton of New York,[17] Wilson of Pennsylvania,[18] and even Madison of Virginia[19] to the inclusion of a Bill of Rights in the original Constitution. When Madison changed his mind and indeed proposed a Bill of

---

[16] See, in general, John Hart Ely, *Democracy and Distrust* (Cambridge, Mass.: Harvard University Press, 1980); idem, "The Wages of Crying Wolf: A Comment on *Roe v. Wade,*" *Yale Law Journal* 82 (1972): 920.

[17] See no. 84, *The Federalist Papers,* ed. Clinton Rossiter (New York: Mentor, 1961).

[18] See Jonathan Elliot, *The Debates in the Several State Conventions on the Adoption of the Federal Constitution* (Washington, D.C., 1836), 2: 434–437, 453–455.

[19] *Ibid.,* 3: 620, 626–627.

Rights in the first meetings of the House of Representatives, he carefully guarded against the unjust inference that the Bill of Rights exhausted the rights enforceable against the federal government by inclusion of the Ninth Amendment;[20] and the assumption of such reserved rights was also appealed to by one or another of the clauses of the Fourteenth Amendment as constraints on state power as well.[21] There is, therefore, no question that both the text and history of the Constitution contemplated enforceable rights beyond those specified in the Bill of Rights, and the most clear-headed constitutional critics of the constitutional right to privacy (namely, John Hart Ely) have clearly acknowledged that their objection to the abortion decisions in particular is not because of text or history, but because they (Ely) hold a political theory (namely, utilitarianism) which objects, in principle, to such a right.[22] This, in my judgment, is precisely *not* to take seriously either constitutional text or history.

Ely defends this move by distinguishing the protection accorded privacy interests by specific provisions of the Fourth Amendment (notably, the search and seizure prohibitions) from the distinguishable interests protected by the constitutional right to privacy.[23] It is certainly true that the constitutional right to privacy is not limited to the interest in informational privacy protected by the Fourth Amendment (abortions, for example, do not usually take place in the privacy of the home), but it is a mistake to think therefore that

[20] See Bernard Schwartz, *The Great Rights of Mankind* (New York: Oxford University Press, 1977), p. 167.

[21] Ely puts particular weight here on the privileges and immunities clause of the Fourteenth Amendment, which, he believes, importantly incorporates the idea of unenumerated fundamental rights from the privileges and immunities clause of Article IV: see Ely, *Democracy and Distrust*, pp. 22–30. The Supreme Court, of course, has based the inference of unenumerated rights on the due process clause of the Fourteenth Amendment: see, e.g., *Roe v. Wade*, 410 U. S. 113 (1973).

[22] For further discussion of Ely's arguments on this point, see Richards, *Toleration and the Constitution*, ch. 8; see also chs. 1 and 10.

[23] See Ely, *Democracy and Distrust*, p. 221, n. 4. Cf. Ely, "Wages of Crying Wolf," pp. 920, 928–930.

constitutional privacy strains the concept of privacy to the conceptual breaking point. The most abstract sense of privacy—freedom from unjust intrusion—includes the distinction between the public and private spheres, and more specific concerns for the control of private information and of choices essential to a private life.[24] Privacy, in the sense of information control, elaborates only one of the strands of this more abstract concept of privacy; other strands of this concept include a sphere of private life immune from state intrusion. We must therefore not dismiss protections of this latter sphere as not "privacy," properly so-called, for that is conceptual nonsense. Rather, we should ask the deeper normative question of whether our constitutional traditions—properly understood— protect such a sphere and to what extent.

In fact, many classical constitutional rights specify such zones of privacy, that is, areas of human life removed from state intrusion. For example, we regard religious belief, practice, and even action (when not violating compelling secular interests) as intrinsically private matters, and yet not because we associate religion with informational privacy (many religious activities take place in public). Rather, our commitment to the right to conscience associates integrity itself with the control of each person over the formation of the ultimate aims of our moral powers (for example, an identity formed in personal relationship to an ethical God). Accordingly, we think of this relationship as not properly a matter of public interest and protect it from a hostile public concern that compromises the moral independence expressed and often perfected in such relationships.

For similar reasons, our constitutional tradition has traditionally extended this private sphere more generally to those highly personal relationships and activities like marriage[25]

[24] See David A. J. Richards, "Privacy," *Collier's Encyclopedia* (New York: Macmillan, 1986), 19: 393–395.
[25] There can be little historical doubt that one such assumed basic human right was the natural right to marriage. For example, Hutcheson's widely read and studied

whose just moral independence requires special protection from a hostile public interest that unjustly compromises the range of thought, self-image, emotional vulnerabilities, sensitivities, and aspirations essential to the role of such relationships and activities in the formation of self expressive of one's moral powers. Such intimate personal relationships—which give play to love, devotion, friendship as organizing themes in self-conceptions of permanent value in living—are among the essential resources of moral independence. Protection from hostile interest thus protects these intimate personal resources, a wholeness of emotion, intellect, and self-image guided by the self-determining moral powers of a free person. Accordingly, the right to form voluntary relationships like marriage was naturally understood as one of the fundamental rights reserved from state power by the Ninth and Fourteenth amendments, and is thus the natural interpretive basis of the elaboration in our law of the constitutional right to privacy.[26]

Criminal prohibitions bearing on the right of constitutional privacy require a heavy burden of justification which can, in principle, be met. There would, I assume, be no constitutional objection to the application of neutral criminal statutes to intrafamilial murders, or wife or husband beatings, or child abuse, no matter how rooted in intimate family life and sexuality; nor should there be any objection to rape laws if

works list, among other fundamental rights, "the natural right each one has to enter into the matrimonial relation with any one who consents": Francis Hutcheson, *A System of Moral Philosophy* [1755] (New York: Augustus M. Kelley, 1968), p. 299. Indeed, there is good historical reason to suppose that this right was thought of as one, nonexclusive example of a more abstract right of voluntary association. Striking evidence of this appears in the lectures of John Witherspoon, a form of which James Madison heard and studied while a student at Princeton. Witherspoon, tracking Hutcheson's list of basic human rights, lists a "right to associate, if he so inclines, with any person or persons, whom he can persuade (not force)—under this is contained the right to marriage": John Witherspoon, *Lectures on Moral Philosophy* (East Brunswick, N. J.: Associated University Presses, 1982), p. 123.

[26] Cf. Kenneth I. Karst, "The Freedom of Intimate Association," *Yale Law Journal* 89 (1980): 624; David A. J. Richards, "Sexual Autonomy and the Constitutional Right to Privacy," *Hastings Law Journal* 30 (1979): 957, and "Unnatural Acts and the Constitutional Right to Privacy," *Fordham Law Review* 45 (1977): 1281.

applicable to married or unmarried sexual intimacies. In these cases, the constitutional burden of justification is met: countervailing rights of persons justify coercive interference into intimate relations.

On the other hand, the principle of the cases elaborating the constitutional right to privacy[27] rests on the vindication of a right of intimate association whose coercive prohibition by state laws cannot satisfy the constitutionally required burden of justification. In *Griswold v. Connecticut*,[28] for example, the state prohibition on the use of contraceptives in marriage limited the basic right of married couples to regulate the form of their sexual lives and their procreative consequences in forming new intimate relations with offspring. Such state prohibitions could not in contemporary circumstances satisfy the constitutional burden of protecting the rights of other persons: on the contrary, legitimate state purposes of population control may thus be advanced. And they could not reasonably be supposed to protect persons from self-destructive harms to self: contraceptive use in marriage has secured to couples the dignity of a deepened freedom and rationality of sexual expression in their intimate personal lives and greater control over their reproductive and other personal aims. Perhaps for the first time in human history, women in general can have personally expressive sexual lives and relationships, unburdened by self-conceptions of mandatory procreative function and duty. In sum, the choice to use contraceptives has been a key exercise of constructive moral powers in the redefinition of personal relationships. Any residual justification of these laws prohibiting contraception appears grounded either on ideals of the necessary link of sex and procreation,[29] or the associated

---

[27] *Griswold v. Connecticut*, 381 U. S. 449 (1958) (contraception use by married couples); *Eisenstadt v. Baird*, 405 U. S. 438 (1972) (contraception use by unmarried); *Stanley v. Georgia*, 394 U. S. 557 (1969) (obscene materials used in home); *Roe v. Wade*, 410 U. S. 113 (1973) (abortion services).

[28] 381 U.S. 449 (1958).

[29] See Augustine, *The City of God* (Harmondsworth: Penguin, 1972), pp. 577–594.

thought that sex without procreation is a kind of homicide.[30] But neither justification can satisfy the constitutionally neutral burden of justification required for laws that directly abridge fundamental rights of the person: such laws cannot be justified to the many reasonable people who do not share these ideals or the associated thought of nonprocreative sex as homicidal.

The elaboration of the right of constitutional privacy in our law thus requires, for its intelligibility, a distinction between forms of public argument which satisfy the constitutional burden required for its abridgment and other forms of argument which cannot meet this burden. The nature and point of this distinction is the same conception of secular purposes explicit in religion clause jurisprudence, namely, the abstract political perspective fundamental to respect for human rights, namely, treating other persons as one would oneself want to be treated, as a person with respect for one's basic demands for those liberties essential to a self-governing person and moral agent.[31] Respect for the liberties essential to our moral autonomy is shown by the limitation of state power to those general goods that all persons, understood as free and equal, could offer and accept as universally applicable constraints on their interpersonal conduct.[32] Such political justification must therefore exclude those conceptions of fact and value that cannot be thus justified: for example, factual claims not justified in the standard empirical ways accessible to all or normative claims resting on sectarian or other

---

[30] St. Thomas elaborates Augustine's conception of the exclusive legitimacy of procreative sex in a striking way. Of the emission of semen apart from procreation in marriage he wrote: "[A]fter the sin of homicide whereby a human nature already in existence is destroyed, this type of sin appears to take next place, for by it the generation of human nature is precluded": T. Aquinas, *On the Truth of the Catholic Faith: Summa Contra Gentiles* (New York: Image, 1956).

[31] See, in general, John Rawls, *A Theory of Justice* (Cambridge, Mass.: Harvard University Press, 1971): Richards, *Toleration and the Constitution.*

[32] See John Rawls, "Social Unity and Primary Goods," in Amartya Sen and Bernard Williams, eds., *Utilitarianism and Beyond* (Cambridge: Cambridge University Press, 1982), pp. 159–185.

perceptions not available to all reasonable persons.[33] The point is not that such conceptions are irrational or nonrational, religious or irreligious, or not of controlling importance in many well-lived lives, but that they do not protect goods that all reasonably accept as the common resources of constructing a valuable life in a community committed to respect for the self-determining rationality of free people. The liberal limitation of state power to such goods—born in the commitment to universal religious toleration[34]—was motivated not by the idea that such goods define what makes a life ultimately meaningful and of value. The idea, rather, is quite the opposite. The pursuit of such goods defines the limits of legitimate state power precisely because they do not themselves define such ultimate questions, but are the all-purpose goods consistent with the kind of interpretive independence on such questions that respect for the inalienable right to conscience requires. Such a limitation of state power is hostile neither to religion nor irreligion, but makes possible a common ground of mutual respect for the inalienable right of persons to adopt incommensurably disparate theories of a good life expressive of the more ultimate religious and philosophical disagreements that respect for this right makes possible and indeed fosters.[35] The liberal proscription on the enforcement at large of such incommensurably disparate theories of a good life thus protects the moral foundations of such mutual respect and the flourishing intellectual, philosophical, and religious diversity it makes possible.[36] Such views cannot justly be enforced at large

[33] I elaborate the requirements of this argument at greater length at pp. 118–121, 133–140, 249–252, in *Toleration and the Constitution;* see also Thomas Nagel, "Moral Conflict and Political Legitimacy," *Philosophy and Public Affairs* 16 (1987): 215.

[34] See, in general, Richards, *Toleration and the Constitution.*

[35] Indeed, leading advocates of universal religious toleration defended it on the religious ground that it freed religion from the corrupting secular incentives of association with state power, and made possible a religious aspiration of respect for persons made in the image of the freedom and rationality of God. See Richards, *Toleration and the Constitution,* pp. 118–121.

[36] Cf. Seymour Martin Lipset, *The First New Nation* (New York: W. W. Norton, 1979), pp. 140–169.

precisely because they are, in Kant's sense, heteronomous:[37] they enforce at large views that many reasonably reject, and thus degrade their just equal liberty to define their ultimate philosophical and moral aims. Mill's harm principle, properly understood, imposes constraints on state power for this reason and to make this political point.[38]

Since the constitutional right to privacy protects the same interests in moral independence protected by the guarantees of religion and speech, unsurprisingly abridgment of the right to privacy—like comparable abridgments of religious liberty or free speech—can only be justified by the necessary and indispensable protection of the claims of persons for the neutral goods all would require to lead their lives as free persons, irrespective of their ideological differences in basic religious or other commitments. Accordingly, the state may justly enforce criminal statutes which enforce ethical principles that, on fair terms to all, protect the interests of adult persons in life, bodily security and integrity, security in institutional relationships and claims arising therefrom, and the interests of children in appropriate conditions of nurture and development. Criminal prohibitions on the use of contraceptives or abortion services or use of obscene materials in the home could not meet this burden of justification: arguments of countervailing rights were either too constitutionally nonneutral or controversial or speculative to satisfy the burden required to abridge such intimately personal sexual matters.

On this view, the constitutional right to privacy arose in our law as the principled protection of a fundamental right of intimate association when traditional justifications for coercive infringements of this right no longer rested on the protection of neutral goods broadly acceptable to the moral consciences of all responsible people, irrespective of their philosophical, religious,

[37] See Immanuel Kant, *Foundations of the Metaphysics of Morals* (New York: Liberal Arts Press, 1959), at *432–436.
[38] I explore this point at greater length in David A. J. Richards, "Kantian Ethics and the Harm Principle: A Reply to John Finnis," *Columbia Law Review* 87 (1987): 457.

and ideological commitments. Indeed, it is precisely because the traditional condemnation appears for this reason unjust that persons require protection by the constitutional right to privacy, for this right enables persons to exercise their independent moral judgment in constructing new kinds of more satisfying and more humane personal and moral relationships.

Constitutional Privacy and Homosexual Love. The principle of constitutional privacy, thus understood, applies to consensual homosexuality because, first, these relationships are a form of the basic right of intimate association, and second, the coercive abridgment of these relationships cannot be justified in the required way. Let me amplify each point, and then address why the traditional moral grounds for the condemnation of homosexuality are today constitutionally suspect. This latter discussion will, I believe, bring out why liberals in general (heterosexual and homosexual) should identify political scapegoating of homosexuals, reflected in public attitudes toward the AIDS crisis, as yet another form of the nativist hatred of political and religious dissent which liberal principles condemn.

First, criminalization of the forms of sexual expression of homosexual love abridges important, exclusive, or primary ways in which many persons in our society naturally feel and express sexual love for one another, voluntarily bond their lives to one another in the intimate relations central to the integrity of their personal lives, and indeed sustain the sexual expression of their personal relationships.[39] Fair social description would underscore the continuities in both the sexual experience and bonding which characterize the place these forms of sexual expression enjoy in the lives of diverse heterosexual and homosexual American couples today, facts attested by the many careful studies which have followed in the

[39] See, for example, Alan P. Bell and Martin S. Weinberg, *Homosexualities* (New York: Simon & Schuster, 1978), pp. 106–115; Philip Blumstein and Pepper Schwartz, *American Couples: Money, Work, Sex* (New York: Morrow, 1983), pp. 237–245.

wake of Kinsey's classic studies.[40] It would blink reality, in this case facts bearing on fundamental constitutional rights, not to give them appropriate weight in elaborating the meaning of abstract background rights in the constitutionally sensitive area of criminal coercion. The attempt by law to isolate and criminally condemn such forms of sexual expression violently deracinates such facts from the lives of the many persons for whom such acts express the meaning for them of their most profound and personally authentic feelings of affection, attachment, and mutual love. This brutal and callous impersonal manipulation of intimate personal life is the same constitutional evil as that condemned by the Supreme Court in disallowing the legitimacy of state control of contraceptive use in sexuality or state control of women's use of their bodies for procreation. Such coercive laws must satisfy a heavy burden of justification; they cannot do so.

Second, statutes that absolutely forbid oral and anal intercourse cannot be justified consistent with acceptably neutral ethical principles applicable to sexual conduct. For example, respect for the developmental rights of immature children would require that various rights, guaranteed to adults, not extend to persons lacking such rational capacities, such as children. Nor is there any objection to the reasonable and neutral regulation of obtrusive sexual solicitation as such or, of course, to forcible forms of intercourse of any kind. In addition, forms of sexual expression would be limited by other ethical principles: principles of not killing, harming, or inflicting gratuitous cruelty (nonmaleficence); principles of paternalism in narrowly defined circumstances; and principles of fidelity.[41]

---

[40] For the continuities in the nature of sexual experience, see especially William H. Masters and Virginia E. Johnson, *Homosexuality in Perspective* (Boston: Little, Brown, 1979). For continuities in both sexual experience and bonding, see Blumstein and Schwartz, *American Couples*.

[41] See, in general, David A. J. Richards, *A Theory of Reasons for Action* (Oxford: Clarendon Press, 1971).

Statutes that absolutely forbid oral and anal intercourse cannot be justified consistent with these principles. Such statutes are not limited to forcible or public forms of sexual intercourse, or sexual intercourse by or with children, but extend to private, consensual acts between adults as well. The argument that such laws are justified by their indirect effect of stopping homosexual intercourse by or with the underaged as absurdly fails to meet the required burden as the claim that absolute prohibition of heterosexual intercourse could be thus justified. There is no reason to believe that homosexuals as a class are any more involved in offenses with the young than heterosexuals.[42] Nor is there any reliable evidence that such laws inhibit children from being naturally homosexual who would otherwise be naturally heterosexual. Sexual preference is settled, largely irreversibly[43] and as a small minority preference,[44] in very early childhood, well before laws of this kind have any effect.[45] If the aim of determining sexual preference by criminal penalty were legitimate, which I

[42] See the classic Kinsey Institute study of sex offenders, Paul H. Gebhard et al., *Sex Offenders* (New York: Bantam, 1965); Martin Hoffman, *The Gay World* (New York: Bantam, 1968), pp. 89–92. In general, seduction of the young appears to be more centered on heterosexual rather than homosexual relations. See Bell and Weinberg, *Homosexualities*, p. 230. One recent study summarizes the pertinent empirical literature on sex offenders against children as follows: "these men are much more likely to have a heterosexual history and orientation than a homosexual one. Contrary to public belief, homosexual adult males rarely molest young male children": Robert L. Geiser, *Hidden Victims: The Sexual Abuse of Children* (Boston: Beacon Press, 1979), p. 75.

[43] See Wainwright Churchill, *Homosexual Behavior Among Males* (New York: Hawthorn, 1967), pp. 283–291; C. A. Tripp, *The Homosexual Matrix* (New York: McGraw-Hill, 1975), p. 251; D. J. West, *Homosexuality* (Chicago: Aldine, 1968), p. 266.

[44] Kinsey states that 4 percent of males are exclusively homosexual throughout their lives: Alfred Kinsey et al., *Sexual Behavior in the Human Male* (Philadelphia: W. B. Saunders, 1948), pp. 650–651.

[45] See, e.g., J. Money and H. Ehrhardt, *Man and Woman, Boy and Girl* (Baltimore: Johns Hopkins University Press, 1972), pp. 153–201. One study hypothesizes that gender identity and sexual object choice coincide with the development of language, i.e., from 18 to 24 months of age. See Money, Hampson and Hampson, "An Examination of Some Basic Sexual Concepts: The Evidence of Human Hermaphroditism," *Bulletin of Johns Hopkins Hospital* 97 (1955): 301. Cf. A. P. Bell, M. S. Weinberg, and S. K. Hammersmith, *Sexual Preference* (Bloomington: Indiana University Press, 1981).

do not concede, that interest could not constitutionally be secured by overbroad statutes which coercively violate the core privacy rights of exclusive homosexuals of all ages and that, in any event, irrationally pursue the state interest.

Other moral principles fail to justify absolute prohibitions on oral and anal sex as such. Such relations are not, for example, generally violent. Thus prohibitory statutes could not be justified by moral principles of nonmaleficence. There is no convincing evidence that all or most such sexual acts as such harm agents or express mental or physical disease[46] so that narrowly drawn paternalistic principles do not here come into proper play.[47] Indeed, if anything, criminalization and associated patterns of discrimination against homosexuals—in contrast to public education—foster health risks,[48] a point to which I shall return in later sections of this essay. And these statutes do not correspond to any just purpose that the state might have in enforcing principles of fidelity: the acts often

---

[46] See *The Wolfenden Report* (New York: Stein & Day, 1963), pp. 31–33; E. Hooker, "The Adjustment of the Male Overt Homosexual," *Journal of Projective Techniques* 21 (1957): 18. Both the American Psychiatric Association and the American Psychological Association no longer regard homosexuality as such as a manifestation of psychological problems: Blumstein and Schwartz, *American Couples*, p. 44.

[47] For example, any general coercive statute directed against sodomy as such, allegedly directed against sexual activity likely to minimize AIDS health risks to the agent, would be grossly overinclusive, condemning the many such acts not subject to such risks at all and other such acts where risks can be reduced by prophylactic measures. Such coercive paternalistic legislation would, even if it could be drawn with appropriate narrowness, still raise substantial issues of justice if its purposes could be more practically and justly achieved by massive public education which properly respects and enhances people's judgment and capacity to decide whether and how they will minimize risks. See Richard D. Mohr, "AIDS, Gay Life, State Coercion," *Raritan* 6 (Summer 1986): 38.

[48] It is the criminalization of sexual activities which leads to their secretive and clandestine nature uninformed of possible health risks, and discourages the kind of candid access to medical information and services which might mitigate the health risks in question: see "The Constitutionality of Laws Forbidding Private Homosexual Conduct," *Michigan Law Review* 72 (1974): 1613, 1631–33. Criminalization and larger patterns of discrimination against homosexuals also render difficult the formation of the kinds of stable relationships which would both minimize health risks and humanely deal with health problems when they occur: see Mohr, "AIDS."

occur in ongoing and longstanding intimate relations, which they may, if anything, stabilize and enrich.

The failure of these laws to satisfy the constitutional burden required for abridgment of constitutional privacy is consistent with the similar failure implicit in the Court's previous applications of constitutional privacy. Like anticontraception laws, these laws coerce people not to engage in nonprocreative sex but do so even more unwarrantably since many homosexual men and women find their exclusive or primary forms of sexual expression in these acts. The interest in autonomy in intimate relations is here at least as strong as that in the reproductive autonomy or abortion decisions or decisions to use obscene materials, and the evidence of harms to the rights of concrete other persons even more controversial and speculative.

One final moral argument has been used to justify a general prohibition on oral and anal sex—the argument invoked by the district court in *Doe*[49] and by the Supreme Court in *Bowers v. Hardwick*[50] as the ultimate ground for the legitimacy of sodomy statutes, namely, "the promotion of morality and decency,"[51] interpreted as an appeal to traditional moral condemnation of certain acts.

A form of public argument is, indeed, necessary to the legitimacy of the criminal law in the United States, but the very elaboration of the constitutional right to privacy consistent with fundamental principles of our constitutional law suggests that not every statement of "morality and decency," which surely could be invoked against all the privacy decisions, is of equal constitutional weight. In fact, all the privacy decisions reflect deep moral controversy within American society over which aspects of our collective moral traditions can and cannot

[49] *Doe v. Commonwealth's Attorney*, 403 F. Supp. 1199 (E. D. Va. 1975), *aff'd without opinion* 425 U. S. 901 (1976) (homosexual acts not protected by constitutional right to privacy).

[50] This argument was endorsed by Justice White, writing for the 5–4 majority of the Supreme Court in *Bowers v. Hardwick*, 106 S. Ct. 2841 (1986).

[51] *Doe v. Commonwealth's Attorney*, 403 F. Supp. 1202.

justly be retained. Our moral practices as a community are not
inextricably homogeneous: on critical reflection, we retain
certain basic principles in them (for example, treating persons
as equals), but change lower order conventions which we come
to believe inconsistent with the reflective ethical core of our
moral and constitutional values. Accordingly, the appeal to
"morality and decency," without more, falsely begs the central
issue in dispute, supposing precisely the kind of homogeneity
in moral values which the general history of Western ethics
and specific history of constitutional privacy belie. It is a valued
and admirable distinction of Western ethics and law that they
have changed, in response to critical reflection on their own
history and to new empirical and normative perspectives.

I have already proposed the kind of ethical principles to
which controversies over proper criminalization appeal, and
explained why criminalization of acts of sexual expression
cannot meet this burden of justification. Why, then, does
hostility to homosexuality enjoy such popular support as a
rallying cry of neoconservatives in a way that opposition to
contraception and even abortion does not? In order to
understand this ugly political fact and the proper attitude to be
taken toward it, we must take seriously the ways in which the
traditional moral conceptions underlying the criminalization of
oral and anal sex reflect a history of false empirical and
dubious moral beliefs that cannot, on reflection, constitutionally enjoy the force of law.

The traditional moral condemnation of oral and anal sex in
our culture may be traced to a number of beliefs: (1) that homosexual forms of such sexual expression undermine, particularly in men, desirable masculine character traits—for example,
courage and self-control;[52] (2) a general conception that sexuality has one proper purpose alone (procreation) and any other
form of sexual expression, disengaged from procreation, is shame-

[52] For the earliest literate statement of this view, see Plato, *Laws*, bk. VIII,
835d–842a.

fully wrong (including contraception use); (3) an empirical belief that prohibitions of homosexual forms of such sexual expression combated natural disasters like earthquakes;[53] (4) a theological misconception that relevant passages in the Old and New Testaments condemned such acts; (5) various empirical beliefs about the inhumanly exceptional choice of sexual propensities, the evil consequences of their exercise to the agent and others (child molestation), their connections with other moral vices, etc.; and (6) a political conception that such acts constitute a form of willful heresy or treason against the stability of social institutions. All these beliefs are, in fact, either factually false or based on moral premises (for example, the sexist premise that sex between men degrades one of them into a woman, or the norm of sex as procreative) that we now reject as not properly enforceable on society at large, and should constitutionally reject as reasonable grounds for the application of coercive sanctions to oral and anal sex as such. Why, then, do people (including the Supreme Court of the United States) isolate homosexuality from their views about contraception and abortion?

In part, this may reflect the simple demographic fact that homosexuality remains and will remain a small minority preference, whereas contraception and abortion pervade American social life at all levels. People can understand the latter, but have little experience with the former. Accordingly, they acknowledge and sometimes accept constitutional principles to protect popular forms of nonprocreative (heterosexual) sex, but fail to see that these principles apply also to less popular forms of nonprocreative (homosexual) sex.

---

[53] See Justinian, Novellae 77 and 141, reprinted in D. Bailey, *Homosexuality and the Western Christian Tradition* (New York and London: Longmans, Green, 1955), pp. 73–75. The issuance of these imperial edicts seems to have been prompted by contemporary earthquakes, floods, and plagues, which Justinian, drawing an analogy to the Sodom and Gomorrah episode, supposed to be caused by homosexual practices: *ibid.*, pp. 76–77. Blackstone similarly cites the Sodom and Gomorrah episode in support of the appropriateness of the death penalty for homosexual acts, indeed suggesting—since God there punished by fire—the special appropriateness of death by burning: W. Blackstone, *Commentaries*, vol. 4, *216.

At a deeper level, this isolation reflects the ancient and modern conception that homosexual forms of oral and anal sex are a form of heresy or treason.[54] Of course, there is no good reason to believe that the legitimacy of such forms of sexual expression destabilizes social cooperation; homosexual relations are and will foreseeably remain the preference of small minorities of the population,[55] who are as committed to principles of social cooperation and contribution as any other group in society at large. Indeed, the very accusation of heresy or treason brings out an important feature of the traditional moral condemnation in its contemporary vestments: it rests no longer on generally acceptable arguments of protection of the rights of persons to neutral goods, but appeals to arguments internal to highly personal, often almost religious decisions about acceptable ways of belief and lifestyle.

The point—the point that makes homosexuals a popular object of social contempt and scorn—is that homosexuals are and must remain exiles from the family. Of course, these perceptions create the thing on which they feed, for they compulsively exile homosexuals from anything resembling family life by denying them child custody or the legal protections of marriage or the antidiscrimination protections

[54] Throughout the Middle Ages, homosexuals were prosecuted as heretics, often being burned at the stake. See Bailey, *Homosexuality*, p. 135. Thus "buggery," one of the names for homosexual acts, derives from a corruption of the name of one heretical group alleged to engage in homosexual practices: *ibid.*, pp. 141, 148–149. For a modern use of treason in this context, see P. Devlin, *The Enforcement of Morals* (London: Oxford University Press, 1965), pp. 1–25. For rebuttal, see H. L. A. Hart, *Law, Liberty, and Morality* (Stanford: Stanford University Press, 1963); also "Social Solidarity and the Enforcement of Morals," *University of Chicago Law Review* 35 (1967): 1.

[55] The original Kinsey estimate that about 4 percent of males are exclusively homosexual throughout their lives is confirmed by comparable European studies. See Paul H. Gebhard, "Incidence of Overt Homosexuality in the United States and Western Europe," in J. M. Livingood, ed., *National Institute of Mental Health Task Force on Homosexuality* (Washington, D. C.: U. S. Government Printing Office, 1972), pp. 22–29. The incidence figure remains stable though many of the European countries do not apply the criminal penalty to consensual adult sex acts of the kind here under discussion: see W. Barnett, *Sexual Freedom and the Constitution* (Albuquerque: University of New Mexico Press, 1973), p. 293.

essential to a secure personal life. But that is the vicious circularity of the neoconservative ideology I am describing. And that is precisely why homosexuals as a group so clearly require protection by the constitutional right to privacy.

Since the traditional moral condemnation of homosexuality must now abandon certain of its essential grounds (beliefs in harm, for example), the abandonment of these grounds must, *pari passu*, deprive the tradition of its constitutional legitimacy as a ground for coercive sanctions. For the tradition now no longer expresses ethical arguments which may fairly be imposed on all persons, but rather perspectives reasonably authoritative only for those internal to the tradition. Enforcement of such perspectives on society at large is, as I have suggested, the functional equivalent of a heresy prosecution:[56] the grounds for prohibition are highly personal ideological or political disagreements among which free persons reasonably disagree; and the continuing force of the prohibitions rests, on examination, not on protection of the rights of persons, but on fears and misunderstandings directed at the alien way of life of a small and traditionally condemned minority, as if, at bottom, the legitimacy of one's way of life requires the illegitimacy of all others. Constitutional toleration, which forbids heresy prosecutions[57] and sharply circumscribes treason prosecutions,[58] must likewise be extended to criminal prohibitions which today have the political force of heresy and treason prosecutions.

Since the criminal prohibition of homosexuality can no longer be acceptably justified, homosexuals have the basic right of moral independence to construct conceptions both of personal relationships and of community in accord with their

---

[56] The English legal scholar, Tony Honore, observed of the contemporary status of the homosexual: "It is not primarily a matter of breaking rules but of dissenting attitudes. It resembles political or religious dissent, being an atheist in Catholic Ireland or a dissident in Soviet Russia": Tony Honore, *Sex Law* (London: Duckworth, 1978), p. 89.

[57] "Heresy trials are foreign to our Constitution," *United States v. Ballard,* 322 U.S. 78, 86 (Douglas, J., writing for the Court).

[58] See U.S. Constitution, Art. III, Sec. 3.

reasoned convictions of permanent value in living, and to present these conceptions as one among the competing pluralistic visions of value in living that enrich the range of the humane imagination of a free people. Hopefully, those conceptions will enrich the social imagination of us all as homosexual couples show us that love is not gender defined, that the relationships of neither men nor women must be frigidly locked into competitive hostility, that the redemptive force of personal love is an inalienable right of the human soul whose needs know not gender.

Human Rights and Public Health

It is at the heart of our contemporary dilemma that these arguments have not yet achieved the level of political and constitutional acceptance that they deserve.[59] It is precisely because homosexuals have not yet been guaranteed the minimal rights of privacy and antidiscrimination that are, as a matter of principle, their due that they are unjustly vulnerable to the abusive use of arguments of public health, including the idea of moral plague (more fully discussed in the next section), and that public-health policies must be subjected to a higher level of scrutiny to insure that they are indeed effective as well as respectful of rights.

It is, of course, a now-notorious fact of American history that arguments of public health (control of venereal disease) were abusively invoked against prostitutes to justify policies of criminalization and quarantine that were, as policies of public health, dangerously ineffective and diverted attention from alternative regulatory policies that better controlled spread of the disease.[60] In effect, progressive reformers committed to

[59] See, in particular, *Bowers v. Hardwick*, 106 S. Ct. 2841 (1986).

[60] See, in general, Allan M. Brandt, *No Magic Bullet: A Social History of Venereal Disease in the United States Since 1880* (New York: Oxford University Press, 1985). On the medicalization of the antiprostitution issue, see *ibid.*, p. 94. See also Allan M.

public health were co-opted to the theretofore unsuccessful moral agenda of the purity leagues, and thus successfully established policies of criminalization and quarantine on what appeared to be neutral secular grounds of public health, but were in fact thinly disguised sectarian moral condemnations of prostitution itself. Recent proposals for the mass quarantine of those with AIDS or who test positive for the AIDS antibody— clearly unjustified as public-health policies since AIDS is not contagious[61]—illustrate the continuing force of such abusive arguments of public health in American public life. We can only guard against them if we insist that conceptions of the legitimate scope of the public-health power satisfy more demanding tests of effectiveness than have hitherto been required. Since the invocation of such public-health power may now plausibly be threatened against conduct arguably protected by the constitutional right to privacy, the time for insisting on such a reexamination is surely exigently at hand.[62] Such higher scrutiny will, in complementary fashion, both better secure respect for rights and lead to more effective public-health policies.

Indeed, there is good reason to believe that no public-health program directed against limiting the AIDS epidemic can be effective if it fails to respect the rights of homosexuals to privacy and antidiscrimination. Sexually active male homosexuals are, of course, the group at highest risk for AIDS in the United States.[63] They stand to profit enormously from effective public-health programs that limit the further spread

---

Brandt, "AIDS: From Social History to Social Policy," *Law, Medicine & Health Care* 14 (1986): 231; Charles E. Rosenberg, "Disease and the Social Order in America: Perceptions and Expectations," *Milbank Quarterly* 64, Supp. 1 (1986): 34.

[61] See, in general, David F. Musto, "Quarantine and the Problem of AIDS," *Milbank Quarterly* 64, Supp. 1 (1986): 97.

[62] For a promising proposal along these lines, see Larry Gostin, "The Future of Communicable Disease Control: Toward a New Concept in Public Health," *Milbank Quarterly* 64, Supp. 1 (1986): 79.

[63] See Mueller, "Epidemiology of the Human Immunodeficiency Virus Infection," pp. 250–252.

of a deadly virus that they would certainly count as a secular harm on any reasonable understanding of the harm principle. All persons (homosexual and heterosexual) have a right to just and effective state programs that protect them from such deadly harms, but male homosexuals—the highest risk group—have the liveliest personal interest in securing this right. Such programs include testing that enables them responsibly to know whether they do or do not test positive for the virus. But homosexuals cannot reasonably be expected to undertake such tests if the results could be used, as they could in half the states of the United States, as evidence to convict them of a criminal wrong, or could be used, as they could in most states, to justify forms of discrimination against them in access to housing, employment, and the like. It is precisely the fact that homosexuals are not guaranteed the rights of privacy and antidiscrimination that are their due that make them vulnerable to forms of unjust victimization with which they may ethically refuse complicity. Good and innocent people, free of any wrongdoing over which the state has legitimate authority, should, of course, not be put in such a dilemma: the choice between reasonable health care and loss of their elementary human rights. But they cannot be condemned for failing to participate in health-care programs that are in their own interest when they reasonably perceive nonparticipation as the necessary price they must pay to preserve their lives from unjust stigma and victimization. The only responsible course is, I believe, to design testing programs that do not put homosexuals to this unjust choice (including ironclad guarantees of confidentiality),[64] and to redouble our efforts to remove the violations of homosexuals' rights to privacy and antidiscrimination that frame the dilemma.

[64] See, in general, Michael J. Barry, Paul D. Cleary, and Harvey V. Fineberg, "Screening for HIV Infection: Risks, Benefits, and the Burden of Proof," *Law, Medicine and Health Care* 14 (1986): 259; Kenneth H. Mayer, "The Clinical Challenges of AIDS and HIV Infection," *Law, Medicine and Health Care* 14 (1986): 281; Lewis H. Kuller and Lawrence A. Kingsley, "The Epidemic of AIDS: A Failure of Public Health Policy," *Milbank Quarterly* 64, Supp. 1 (1986): 56.

There is one public-health strategy—namely, massive public education in ways of avoiding transmission of the virus, including use of condoms—that should enjoy a high priority on grounds both of respect for rights and effectiveness. Surely, public education in realistic health risks and ways of avoiding them treat persons, including homosexuals, as responsible moral agents, bringing to their attention how they might, consistent with the larger framework of their aims and purposes, structure their sexual lives to minimize health risks to themselves and others that they do and would want reasonably to avoid. Such a public policy has the notable political virtue—familiar from campaigns of public education about cigarette smoking—that it avoids making controversially paternalistic judgments about the values people find in living, rather limiting itself to important issues of fact that persons themselves would reasonably use in adopting strategies better to pursue their own ends and larger vision of value in living. There are very strong reasons of justice, rooted in our society's longstanding failure to respect the rights of privacy and antidiscrimination of homosexuals, why we should, as a matter of public policy, resist—to the maximum extent feasible[65]— imposing such judgments on homosexuals. For the very injustice to which they have been subjected is that aims essential to their emotional and spiritual integrity have been traduced as immorally harmful or diseased when such condemnation failed to take seriously the ways in which persons could and did integrate homosexual preference into fulfilled and ethically responsible lives.[66] In effect, the injustice rested on the degrading assumption that a life lived in accord with homosexual preference reflects either rational incapacity

---

[65] For forms of public-health orders that might square with these requirements, see Larry Gostin, "The Future of Communicable Disease Control," pp. 91–95; see also Institute of Medicine, *Mobilizing Against AIDS*, pp. 139–145.

[66] On the abusive use of paternalistic arguments along these lines, see David A. J. Richards, *Sex, Drugs, Death and the Law: An Essay on Human Rights and Overcriminalization* (Totowa, N. J.: Rowman & Littlefield, 1982), pp. 57–61, 112–116.

or diminished capacity because it pursues a life intrinsically harmful or diseased. If we now see that such paternalistic judgments masked controversially ideological judgments of value in living that cannot justly be enforced through public law in a liberal society, we must see that their insult to the moral integrity of homosexuals is their degradation of the rational powers of homosexuals as persons. A group that has historically suffered from the enforcement through public law of such unjustly debilitating assumptions is surely owed respect for their rational powers to make appropriate judgments about health risks to which they are peculiarly subject, and not to be subjected to any further insult about their capacity to know, identify, and pursue their interests and to find value in living a fulfilled and ethically responsible life.

It is, however, symptomatic of our dilemma that the most just and effective public-health policy—massive public education—should have been the least well funded by the federal government and often most politically controversial.[67] It is the very political virtue of this policy (namely, its candid respect for the reasonable judgment of the groups most afflicted by the virus) that is the focus of its neoconservative opposition, for they are absorbed not by mitigating the spread of a deadly virus but by not legitimating sexual conduct they regard as immoral. If the choice were between saving lives and not legitimating immorality, they would prefer the latter, a preference made with tragic clarity in the continuing refusal either to supply clean needles to IV drug users or to undertake massive education for such users in avoiding health risks.[68] This view makes sense not on the basis of any merely statistical showing that public education would increase the number of "immoral" acts (which may well be false and demonstrably

---

[67] See Larry Gostin, "The Nucleus of a Public Health Strategy to Combat Aids," *Law, Medicine and Health Care* 14 (1986): 226; Leon Eisenberg, "The Genesis of Fear: AIDS and the Public's Response to Science," *idem*, pp. 247–248.

[68] See Eisenberg, "The Genesis of Fear," pp. 247–248; Ginzburg, "Intravenous Drug Abusers and HIV Infections," pp. 270–271.

false), but on the normative assumption of interference with the natural punishment for immorality, that is, the idea of moral plague to which I next turn.

The Idea of Moral Plague

The ethics and law of the West are, I have suggested, peculiarly self-critical, bringing to bear on their contemporary self-understandings tools of historiography, empirical science, and ethical reflection that enable them to select strands of their traditions that respect liberty of conscience and reject religious persecution, or respect equal liberties and reject slavery and the subjection of women, or respect an abstract right of personal privacy and reject traditional refusals to extend the right to contraception or abortion or homosexual relations. We self-consciously carry forward ethical and legal values that are the cumulative product of critical reflection on our history and its meaning in contemporary circumstances, and it is a constitutive feature of the self-reflective process that histori-cally familiar assumptions, once supposed fundamental to social order (for example, the inferiority of women), are debunked as factually and normatively unsustainable. We come correspondingly to define our contemporary moral responsibilities against a background of now-discredited traditional assumptions. It is now morally irresponsible to act on assumptions merely because our ancestors deemed them unquestionable.

These issues are, I believe, crucially at stake in the social construction of the AIDS epidemic as a plague on the model of William McNeill's *Plagues and Peoples*.[69] It is, of course, true that human history has been crucially shaped by deadly

---

[69] William H. McNeill, *Plagues and Peoples* (Garden City, N. Y.: Anchor, 1977); see also Frederick F. Cartwright, *Disease and History* (London: Hart-Davis, MacGibbon, 1972).

plagues in McNeill's sense, that is, epidemics of microparasites that devastated whole peoples with pivotal consequences for the direction of human history. The conquest of the Amerindians by the Spanish conquistadors could not have taken place with the ease or on the scale or with the consequences that it did had not an epidemic of microparasites to which the Amerindians, unlike the Spaniards, were not immune effectively wiped out some 95 percent of the indigenous peoples.[70]

It is, however, fundamental to this historical process not only that many people die, but that the people who survive interpret these events in terms of the idea of moral plague, namely, that the deaths are a just punishment for wrongdoing or failure. Such beliefs thus demoralize the culture of the dead and dying, and correspondingly inspirit the culture immune to the plague.[71] A natural fact, namely, spread of a virus to people not immune to the virus from a people who are immune, is interpretively moralized with important independent consequences for the ultimate direction of human history.

The idea of moral plague is a more primitive metaphor of illness than the essentially romantic and individualistic metaphors (TB and cancer) explored to such telling effect by Susan Sontag.[72] It arises not from a historical moment in the evolution of one culture's ideals of romantic individualism against oppressive social convention, but from unspeakably tragic and scientifically inexplicable facts common to all cultures until very recently in human history.[73] Enormous numbers of people in a society (lovers, friends, family, leaders, etc.) die from a mysterious disease whose origins and mechanisms are not understood at all, nor are any scientifically reliable steps available to control or cure the deadly disease. The society experiences collective powerlessness before unspeakably tragic losses, and the overwhelming hu-

---

[70] McNeill, *Plagues and Peoples*, p. 190.
[71] *Ibid.*, pp. 183–184.
[72] Sontag, *Illness as Metaphor*.
[73] See, e.g., McNeill, *Plagues and Peoples*, pp. 190–191.

man needs of persons to understand and make sense and assert control universally lead to the idea of moral plague: the deaths are not pointless and inexplicable and without remedy, but can be understood and brought within our control as condign punishments for some wrong or failure. Since the punishment is collective, the society must identify and rectify the wrong for which it is collectively responsible, which may be the wrong of its leader (pharaoh's refusal to free the Israelites, or Oedipus's parricide and incest) or of some offending subgroup (killing Jews in the Middle Ages in response to the bubonic plagues[74]) or of the society itself for violating applicable norms (for example, the norms of the covenant with God of ancient Israel interpreted and vindicated by his prophets). Since disease assumedly reflects wrongdoing, often substitutive punishments are offered (the flagellants in the Middle Ages[75]). Sometimes the justice of certain such punishments will be questioned (Job), but the challenge assumes the framework of the idea of moral plague, and raises ultimate questions about the nature of God and ethics within that framework. Since the operative metaphor for the plague is punishable moral pollution, the remedies standardly are a kind of quarantine of the contamination,[76] including cleansing the society of the pollution by removal from society (exile of Oedipus, segregation of lepers).

Ideas of moral plague and related theological explanations of natural events never, of course, occupied the entire field of human thinking. Primitive farmers knew that they had to plant and care for their fields if there was to be a successful crop, but they also concurrently entertained theological beliefs about how related natural events bearing on a successful crop (for example, the weather) might be secured by the use of rituals and prayer. Conceptions of scientific and moral causality were concurrent ways of explaining and controlling events in the

[74] See Cartwright, *Disease and History*, p. 46.
[75] *Ibid.*, p. 47.
[76] On the quarantine of lepers, see Musto, "Quarantine and the Problem of AIDS," pp. 99–101.

world, and one or the other was emphasized depending on human needs for both explanation and control.[77] We may say that, in the area of the deadly epidemics that McNeill calls plagues, the lack of any reliable models of scientific causality or control led to the hegemonic dominance of the idea of moral plague in this area until quite recently in human history.

The idea of moral plague is as powerfully important an idea in the religion and literature of Western culture as any other culture, and we need to be clear that the conditions that gave the idea a sense and point (namely, indiscriminate and inexplicable mass deaths from an unknown and uncontrollable disease) have been removed only recently by the discovery of sound explanations (the germ theory of disease) and, over time, corresponding methods of prevention and cure. These novelties both of explanation and control have removed the context that gave a general hegemonic force to the idea of moral plague, because for the first time in human history reliable models of scientific causality could and did occupy this field.[78] The point is not that religious thinking as such is now outmoded, but that a certain form of religious explanation (the idea of moral plague) no longer is reasonably supposed by religious and nonreligious people alike to be true to fact or capable of responding to our practical needs for prediction and control; rather, scientific models of causality now occupy this field since they better meet our needs for both explanation and for the prevention, diagnosis, and cure of disease. Indeed, to the extent the idea of moral plague assumes a natural retributive order of disease and death, the general idea must reasonably be and is rejected by modern societies, like the United States, committed to the role of modern medicine in

[77] See, in general, Robin Horton, "African Traditional Thought and Western Science," in Bryan R. Wilson, ed., *Rationality* (New York: Harper & Row, 1970), pp. 131–171; Robin Horton, "Tradition and Modernity Revisited," in Martin Hollis and Steven Lukes, eds., *Rationality and Relativism* (Oxford: Basil Blackwell, 1982), pp. 201–260.
[78] See, in general, McNeill, *Plagues and Peoples*, pp. 208–257.

asserting human control over the incidence of disease. We would not, in general, reject the role of the state in public-health policy because that policy has ended diseases like smallpox, measles, and polio, and thus upset the natural retributive order that those diseases reflect. To the contrary, we accept the role of the state in this area as securing a general good (health) that we all reasonably want, and construe this end as consistent with the wide range of more ultimate and often incommensurable religious and philosophical values we find in living a fulfilled and ethical life.

But if there is no continuing general force, as a matter of political principle, in the idea of moral plague, the idea can, I believe, enjoy no more localized political force. Consider the popular conception of AIDS as the gay plague.[79]

First, the conception is willfully nescient of the facts: AIDS is not a disease intrinsic to homosexual sexuality as such. It is a virus probably first transmitted to humans from animals in Africa[80] and that appears to be largely transmitted in Africa heterosexually.[81] It is a contingent historical fact that the virus was introduced into the United States through homosexual relations and was thus transmitted through homosexual sex to sexually active male homosexuals.[82] It is factually grotesque to suppose that homosexual sexuality as such is diseased, or that heterosexual sexuality is naturally immune from the disease. Indeed, the idea of AIDS as the gay plague is an abuse of the idea of moral plague itself, which has its natural home in the arena of indiscriminate mass deaths from an inexplicable and uncontrollable disease; but AIDS is, of course, not contagious, and its origins and mode of transmission are now understood.[83]

Second, the conception of AIDS as the gay plague

---

[79] See, in general, Eisenberg, "Genesis of Fear."

[80] See Institute of Medicine, *Mobilizing Against AIDS*, pp. 71–72.

[81] *Ibid.*, pp. 16–18.

[82] For a plausible chronology, see Randy Shilts, *And the Band Played On* (New York: St. Martin's Press, 1987).

[83] See, in general, Institute of Medicine, *Mobilizing Against AIDS*.

illegitimately seeks to transmute highly controversial sectarian moral objections to homosexuality as such into a superficially more plausible and appealing secular argument about control of deadly disease. The claims have, however, nothing in common.

As I earlier showed, the sectarian moral objections to homosexuality as such can no more justly be enforced through public law than the comparable objections to the sale and use of contraceptives or to access to abortion services. There is no compelling secular argument that could justify the continuing criminalization of homosexual sexuality as such.

Certainly, health risks to some homosexuals from certain forms of sexual intercourse cannot justify prohibition of homosexual sexual intimacy as such which often does not involve health risks any more than the widespread presence of venereal disease in the heterosexual population could justify the prohibition of all heterosexual intimacy; indeed, failure to guarantee homosexuals their human rights to privacy and antidiscrimination has, if anything, fostered health risks. Criminalization and employment risks naturally make it less reasonable for homosexuals to form the kinds of stable relationships that would both minimize health risks and humanely deal with health problems when they occur,[84] and hardly offer them anything even approximating a fair equivalent to the cultural supports for stable personal relations that surround and indeed sanctify heterosexual relations; and criminalization and discrimination, as I earlier argued, discourage the kind of candid access to medical information and services that might enhance people's judgment and capacity to decide how best to mitigate health risks and profit from health programs that are clearly in their interests.[85] In short, a fair concern for public health would, if anything,

[84] See, in general, Mohr, "AIDS" p. 38.
[85] See "Constitutionality of Laws Forbidding Private Homosexual Conduct."

bolster the case for recognizing the rights of homosexuals to privacy and antidiscrimination.

The conception of AIDS as the gay plague illegitimately elides the moral and health-care issues because it reads these issues through the prism of a sectarian commitment to a localized version of the idea of moral plague, namely, that the immorality of homosexuality is justly punishable by death. The ugly consequence of this commitment is that health measures effectively concerned to limit or cure the disease must be morally suspect interventions into the natural retributive order of moralized diseases. That is, of course, not the reasonable health-care policies we have a right to demand and expect in a secular society but the ugly distortion of health-care policy by politically illegitimate moralism historically prefigured by America's failure to adopt effective health policies to control venereal disease and instead moralistically to oppress prostitutes.[86]

Many ordinary Americans do not know or attend to the facts about the transmission of AIDS, and they are not confident about the rights of homosexuals to privacy and antidiscrimination. The idea that AIDS is the gay plague—a factually and morally indefensible view—has achieved the populist currency that it has in this country because our national leadership has been so morally irresponsible in both its failures adequately to fund and engage in massive public education and its failure to support and secure the human rights of homosexuals to privacy and antidiscrimination. It is one thing for some ordinary Americans to take the views they do. It is quite another for an intellectual leader to condemn crash programs for an AIDS vaccine, querying: "Are they aware that in the name of compassion they are giving social sanction to what can only be described as brutish degradation?"[87] Or for the Justice Department to issue in June 1986 a decision that held it

[86] See, in general, Eisenberg, "Genesis of Fear"; Brandt, "AIDS."
[87] The statement was made by Norman Podhoretz, and is cited in Eisenberg, "Genesis of Fear," p. 245.

permissible for employers to bar AIDS patients or those
infected with the virus from work.[88] Or for the Supreme Court
of the United States to engage in the shallow appeal to
unreasoned populist moralism of *Bowers v. Hardwick.*[89] Such
public persons have a corresponding public responsibility not
to appeal to populist fears, but to cultivate the standards of
public reason that make a people worthy of the responsibilities
of democratic government, extending to all persons, on fair
terms, our basic principles of just and good government.
Instead, the Justice Department's decision, for example,
flouted the repeated statements by government scientists, on
the basis of considerable epidemiologic and biological evidence, that the disease was not casually transmitted; and the
Supreme Court abandoned any coherent attempt to explain
why basic principles of an independent private life, fully
extended to heterosexuals despite populist moralistic objections to the contrary, are not extended on fair and equal terms
to homosexuals.[90] Leadership in a democratic society requires
more intelligence, courage, and integrity than these sorry
performances, which, in effect, appeal to the lowest common
denominator of populist fear as the measure of responsible
government and thus feed the forces of hysteria and
unreason.[91] If our leaders will not debunk for us our factual
ignorance and our normative myopia, we are left as a people to
the lowest level of credulity, ignorance, and fear—the miasma
in which the idea of moral plague today politically flourishes.
We thus degrade the ethics of public responsibility required by
our commitment to constitutional government under the rule
of law.

We have outgrown our human need for the idea of moral
plague, an idea rooted in our long historical powerlessness

[88] On the Justice Department ruling, see *New York Times*, June 23 and 27, 1986.
[89] 106 S. Ct. 2841 (1986).
[90] See, in general, Richards, "Constitutional Legitimacy."
[91] See Ronald Bayer, "AIDS, Power, and Reason," *Milbank Quarterly* 64, Supp. 1
(1986): 168.

before deadly epidemic microparasites. Of course, not all beliefs that we outgrow must necessarily be rejected: harmless superstitions (like not having a floor marked 13 on buildings) can be retained without regret or guilt. But the idea of moral plague is not harmless in this way. To the contrary, it is deeply harmful because it falsely moralizes issues of life-threatening disease and obfuscates clear thinking about the essential issues of respect for human rights and public health. Sontag's analysis is here pertinent:

> My point is that illness is *not* a metaphor, and that the most truthful way of regarding illness—and the healthiest way of being ill—is one most purified of, most resistant to, metaphoric thinking . . . It is toward an elucidation of these metaphors, and a liberation from them, that I dedicate this inquiry.[92]

We can perhaps understand and even excuse our ancestors' use of the conceptual paradigm of moral plague, though we can object, as some of them did,[93] to some of the clearly unjust uses to which ignorant and intolerant people put the paradigm. We can perhaps excuse their commitment to the general paradigm because we can, within limits, not hold them responsible for failing to know or ascertain the scientific facts of the transmission of the epidemic diseases that they were confronted with. Our ethical and political situation is, however, different. We know these facts, and we also have reason to know that the idea of moral plague is, for us, a pernicious *conceptual anachronism*,[94] an idea that retains localized political force for us in arenas (AIDS as the gay plague) where it demonstrably threatens injustice. Our ethical and political responsibilities are therefore different; the political use of the

---

[92] Sontag, *Illness as Metaphor*, p. 3.

[93] For example, Pope Clement VI objected to the persecution of Jews during the bubonic plague: Cartwright, *Disease and History*, p. 46.

[94] By a conceptual anachronism, I mean a concept that may once have been excusably used by reasonable people but no longer is.

idea of moral plague is today a morally inexcusable failure of elementary standards of intellectual and ethical responsibility.

To understand the threatened injustice, we need to recall our earlier discussion that homosexuality is today essentially a kind of political, social, and moral dissent on a par with the best American traditions of dissent and even subversive advocacy. The heresy or treason of homosexuals is their rejection of heterosexual family life, a commitment so central to the moral integrity of life's having a meaning for most Americans that homosexuals, as a class, are the ultimate rebels against essential values in living. We can see the political force of these attitudes in the way they equate a homosexual teacher with homosexual seduction of their children, or in the way they transform the heart-rending tragedy of the deaths of many young homosexual men in the AIDS crisis into an aggressive attack by homosexuals on them and their children, requiring isolation of children with AIDS, who did not contract the disease sexually, from public schools.[95] The imaginative transformations here are revealing as they create aggressors out of victims, as they invert moral reality to serve ideological needs under perceived threat from these heretics against the family.

We know enough about the social history of the idea of moral plague to know that it has familiarly been used as a tool of cultural purification of outcast heretics to traditional moral values (for example, Jews in the Middle ages; prostitutes in the drive against venereal disease). The idea of moral plague enjoys the force that it does in contemporary American society because it supplies a conveniently obfuscating metaphor of moralized disease that lends a patina of public-health justification to what is essentially a kind of heresy persecution of homosexuals as moral heretics to the family. It is precisely because this is the political reality that we must liberate

---

[95] See Dorothy Nelkin and Stephen Hilgartner, "Disputed Dimensions of Risk: A Public School Controversy over AIDS," *Milbank Quarterly* 64, Supp. 1 (1986): 118.

ourselves from this pernicious metaphor in service of traditional liberal principles that must protect dissenting ways of life from the worst American impulses of repressive nativism, which find today in homosexuality what they found before in the family planning of Sanger, or the atheism of Darwin, or the socialism of Debs, or the Marxist advocacy of the American Communist Party.

The social history of the idea of moral plagues reveals, as I earlier noted, a characteristic use to justify the moral superiority of peoples who survive plagues and the demoralized sense of failure of peoples who do not (for example, the Amerindians). That moral world is, as matter of general principle, dead for us, for we see it as moralizing natural facts that do not justly deserve the weight historically accorded them. Indeed, we regret and deplore the moral mentality that could so easily morally blame the victims of tragic facts of disease and death.

That moral world retains a localized force in the idea of AIDS as the gay plague. But it is no less unjust there than it is in general. Indeed, it is more unjust, since we make ad hoc use of the idea not merely as a moralizing rationale for our survival and their deaths, but in the self-conscious service of a wholly illegitimate attempt, so I have argued, to demoralize the just claims of homosexuals for their minimal human right to conduct a morally independent private life on fair terms. Homosexuals have, of course, only very recently achieved any measure of moral emancipation from the false factual and normative views that have traditionally denied them personal or political respect for aims essential to the integrity of a fulfilled personal and ethical life, and the localized idea of moral plague is a political strategy directed at demoralizing and retarding this emancipation. But it does so on the basis of distortion of fact and moral obfuscation of the essential issues of human rights and public health.

The idea of moral plague, like the idea of slavery and the subjection of women, is unworthy of us, and it is ethically irresponsible to give the idea any weight in our political lives. We should learn from the social history of plagues that we cannot safely or ethically retain the idea of moral plagues, which corrupts and degrades our traditions of constitutional civility, of toleration, and of ethical decency.

* This article profited from the advice of Donald Levy and from the generous support of the New York University School of Law Filomen D'Agostino and Max E. Greenberg Faculty Research Fund.

method of using blood products HBV vaccine
making does not
transmitt HIV

P. 87. 92, ...